Pernicious Anemia: Everything You Need to Know About the Disease Including Signs and Symptoms, Causes, Treatment and more

Gaby Alez

The role of the book within our culture is changing. The change is brought on by new ways to acquire & use content, the rapid dissemination of information and real-time peer collaboration on a global scale. Despite these changes one thing is clear--"the book" in it's traditional form continues to play an important role in learning and communication. The book you are holding in your hands utilizes the unique characteristics of the Internet -- relying on web infrastructure and collaborative tools to share and use resources in keeping with the characteristics of the medium (user-created, defying control, etc.)--while maintaining all the convenience and utility of a real book.

Contents

Articles

Overview of the Disease

Pernicious anemia

Pernicious anemia	
Classification and external resources	
ICD-10	D 51.0 [1]
ICD-9	281.0 [2]
MedlinePlus	000569 [3]
eMedicine	med/1799 [4]
MeSH	D000752 [5]

Pernicious anemia (or pernicious anemia - also known as **Biermer's anemia**, **Addison's anemia**, or **Addison–Biermer anemia**) is one of many types of the larger family of megaloblastic anemias. It is caused by loss of gastric parietal cells, and subsequent inability to absorb vitamin B_{12}.

Usually seated in an atrophic gastritis, the autoimmune destruction of gastric parietal cells leads to a lack of intrinsic factor. Since the absorption from the gut of normal dietary amounts of vitamin B_{12} is dependent on intrinsic factor, the loss of intrinsic factor leads to vitamin B_{12} deficiency. While the term 'pernicious anemia' is sometimes also incorrectly used to indicate megaloblastic anemia due to *any* cause of vitamin B_{12} deficiency, its proper usage refers to that caused by atrophic gastritis, parietal cell loss, and lack of intrinsic factor only.

The loss of ability to absorb vitamin B_{12} is the most common cause of adult vitamin B_{12} deficiency. Such a loss may be due to pernicious anemia (with loss of intrinsic factor) or to a number of other conditions which decrease production of gastric acid, which also plays a part in absorption of vitamin B_{12} from foods.

Historically, pernicious anemia (PA) was generally detected only after it became "clinical" (caused an overt disease state) and the anemia was well-established, i.e. liver stores of B_{12} had been depleted. The "pernicious" aspects of the disease were peripheral nerve damage and - prior to the discovery of treatment - a prognosis as poor and certain as that of leukemia before it could be treated. However, in the time since elucidation of the cause of the disease, modern tests which specifically target B_{12} absorption can be used to diagnose the disease before it becomes clinically apparent. In such cases, the disease may be diagnosed and treated without the patient ever becoming ill.

Replacement of vitamin stores does not correct the defect in absorption from loss of intrinsic factor, that technically defines the disease. A person who has pernicious anemia defined by inability to absorb vitamin B_{12} in this way, will have it for the remainder of his or her life. However, unless the patient has sustained permanent peripheral nerve damage before treatment, regular B_{12} replacement will keep pernicious anemia in check, with no further damage.

Signs and symptoms

Pernicious anemia presents insidiously, and many of the signs and symptoms are due to anemia itself, where anemia is present. While it may consist of the triad of paraesthesias, sore tongue and weakness, this is not the chief symptom complex. The patient may complain of fatigue, depression, forgetfulness, difficulty concentrating, low-grade fevers, nausea and gastrointestinal symptoms (heartburn), weight loss. Because PA may affect the spinal cord, the patient may also complain of impaired urination, loss of sensation in the feet, unsteady gait, weakness and clumsiness. Anemia may cause tachycardia (rapid heartbeat) and cardiac murmurs, along with a waxy pallor. In severe cases, the anemia may cause evidence of congestive heart failure.

Long term complications may include gastric cancer and carcinoids.

Many signs and symptoms are attributed to pernicious anemia:

- Fatigue, low blood pressure, rapid heart rate, high blood pressure, pallor, depression, muscle weakness and shortness of breath (known as 'the sighs')
- Difficulty in proprioception
- Mild cognitive impairment, including difficulty concentrating and sluggish responses, colloquially referred to as cognitive dysfunctionlbrain fog
- Neuropathic pain
- Frequent diarrhea
- Paresthesias, such as pins and needles sensations or numbness in fingers or toes, due to B_{12} deficiency affecting nerve function
- Jaundice due to impaired formation of blood cells
- Glossitis (swollen red tongue) due to B_{12} deficiency
- May present with hyperthyroidism or hypothyroidism
- Personality or memory changes

A complication of severe chronic PA is subacute combined degeneration of spinal cord, which leads to distal sensory loss (posterior column), absent ankle reflex, increased knee reflex response, and extensor plantar response.

Causes

Most commonly (in temperate climates), the cause for impaired binding of vitamin B_{12} by intrinsic factor is autoimmune atrophic gastritis, in which autoantibodies are directed against parietal cells (resulting in their loss), as well as against the intrinsic factor itself (rendering it unable to bind vitamin B_{12}).

Less frequently, loss of parietal cells may simply be part of a widespread atrophic gastritis of nonautoimmune origin, such as that frequently occurring in elderly people affected with long-standing chronic gastritis of any cause (including *Helicobacter pylori* infection).

Forms of vitamin B_{12} deficiency other than pernicious anemia must be considered in the differential diagnosis of megaloblastic anemia. For example, a B_{12} deficient state which causes megaloblastic anemia and which may be mistaken for classical pernicious anemia, may be caused by infection with the tapeworm *Diphyllobothrium latum*, possibly due to the parasite's competition for vitamin B_{12}.

A similar disorder involving impaired B_{12} absorption can also occur following gastric removal (gastrectomy) or gastric bypass surgery, especially the Roux-en-Y bypass. In this procedure, the stomach is separated into two sections, one a very small pouch for holding small amounts of food, and the other, the remainder of the stomach, which is resultingly nonfunctional. Therefore, the mucosal cells are no longer available, nor is the required intrinsic factor. This results in inadequate GI absorption of B_{12}, and may result in a syndrome indistinguishable from pernicious anemia. Gastric bypass or gastrectomy patients must take B_{12} as in treatment of pernicious anemia: either oral megadoses, or B_{12} by injection.

Pathophysiology

Vitamin B_{12} cannot be produced by the human body, and must be obtained from the diet. Normally, dietary vitamin B_{12} is absorbed by the body in the small bowel only when it is bound by the intrinsic factor (IF) produced by parietal cells of the gastric mucosa. Pernicious anemia is thought to occur when the body's immune system mistakenly targets the intrinsic factor, with a loss of parietal cells. Insufficient IF results in insufficient absorption of the vitamin. Although the normal body stores three to five years' worth of vitamin B_{12} in the liver, the usually undetected autoimmune activity in one's gut over a prolonged period of time leads to vitamin B_{12} depletion and the resulting anemia. Inhibition of DNA synthesis in red blood cells results in the formation of large, fragile megaloblastic erythrocytes.

Diagnosis

The insidious nature of the disease, and the fact that there is no single definitive test for pernicious anemia, may mean that a diagnosis is delayed. Pernicious anemia is suspected when the patient's blood smear shows large, fragile, immature erythrocytes (megaloblasts). The Schilling test is no longer widely available, and the other main diagnostic signpost of low levels of serum B_{12} cannot be relied upon, as sufferers can have high levels of serum B_{12} and still have pernicious anemia. Blood and urine tests for methylmalonic acid may indicate a B_{12} deficiency, even though serum B_{12} is within the normally-acceptable range. Serum B_{12} is not necessarily an indicator of efficient use by the body, in the muscles, for example.

A diagnosis of pernicious anemia first requires demonstration of megaloblastic anemia (through a full blood count) which evaluates the mean corpuscular volume (MCV), as well the mean corpuscular hemoglobin concentration (MCHC). Pernicious anemia is identified with a high MCV and a normal MCHC (that is, it is a macrocytic, normochromic anemia). Ovalocytes are also typically seen on the blood smear, and a pathognomonic feature of megaloblastic anemias (which include pernicious anemia and others) is hypersegmented neutrophils.

Pernicious anemia can also be diagnosed by evaluating its direct cause, vitamin B_{12} deficiency, by measuring B_{12} levels in serum. A Schilling test can then be used to distinguish pernicious anemia from other causes of vitamin B_{12} deficiency (notably malabsorption).

The diagnosis of atrophic gastritis Type A should be confirmed by gastroscopy and stepwise biopsy. Approximately 90% of individuals with PA have antibodies for parietal cells; however, only 50% of all individuals in the general population with these antibodies have pernicious anemia.

Treatment

Main article: Vitamin B12

The treatment of pernicious anemia varies from country to country and from area to area. There is no permanent cure for pernicious anemia, although repletion of vitamin B_{12} should be expected to result in a cessation of anemia-related symptoms, a halt in neurological deterioration, and (in cases where neurological problems not advanced) neurological recovery and a complete and permanent remission of all symptoms, so long as B_{12} is supplemented. Repletion of B_{12} can be accomplished in a variety of ways.

The most accessible and inexpensive method of repletion is through dietary supplementation, in the form of oral or sublingual B_{12} tablets. B_{12} supplements are widely available at supermarkets, health food stores, and drug stores, though quality and cost may vary. In some countries, the cobalamin preparation may be available only via prescription. Doctors can prescribe cobalamin tablets that contain doses higher than what is commercially available.

It is reportedWikipedia:Avoid weasel words that many patients die within 7 days of no treatment while in a severe symptomatic state[citation needed].

A 2003 study found that oral and sublingual B_{12} were absorbed equally well in a group of patients with very low B_{12}. In this study, 22% of the subjects that agreed to undergo the test (5 of 23), had abnormal Schilling tests, but showed no difference in treatment levels from the other subjects. When oral tablets are used to treat PA, higher-than-normal doses may be needed. The efficacy of using high dose B_{12}

tablets to treat ordinary PA (i.e. anemia due to atrophic gastritis) is well established. Oral supplementation allows B_{12} to be absorbed in places other than the terminal ileum (where B_{12} absorption usually takes place). A 2006 study found that oral B_{12} repletion has the potential to be as effective as injections.

However, if oral and sublingual repletion of B_{12} is inadequate, the patient may require B_{12} injections, which are usually given once a month, bypassing the need for gastrointestinal absorption altogether. Eventually, the patient may be able to do this at home. Cobalamin (one of the forms of B_{12}) is usually injected into the patient's muscle (intramuscular or IM) using cyanocobalamin (the United States, Canada and most European countries) or hydroxocobalamin (Australia and the U.K.). The injections will typically need to be given for the remainder of the patient's life. The frequency of injections varies by country and health care practitioner, and may be as infrequent as once every three months in some countries. The most common complaint by members of the Pernicious Anaemia Society is that patients have different needs, with some patients needing more frequent injections than others. Some medical professionalsWikipedia:Avoid weasel words believe that subcutaneous injections are more effective than intramuscular injections, [citation needed] but the evidence for this is currently unclear.

There are other methods of administering B_{12}, including nasal sprays and behind-the-ear patches. One small study from 1997, with six participants, found that intranasal delivery of B_{12} led to increases in plasma cobalamin as high as eight times a given patient's baseline measurement. Further investigation of these delivery methods is needed.

History

The British physician Thomas Addison first described the disease in 1849, from which it acquired the common name of Addison's anemia. In 1907, Richard Clarke Cabot reported on a series of 1200 patients with PA. Their average survival was between one and three years. Dr. William Bosworth Castle performed an experiment whereby he ingested raw hamburger meat and regurgitated it after an hour, and subsequently fed it to a group of ten patients. [citation needed] A control group were fed untreated raw hamburger meat. The former group showed a disease response whereas the latter group did not. This was not a sustainable practice, but it demonstrated the existence of an 'intrinsic factor' from gastric juice.

Pernicious anemia was a fatal disease before about the year 1920, when George Whipple suggested raw liver as a treatment. The first workable treatment for pernicious anemia began when Whipple made a discovery in the course of experiments in which he bled dogs to make them anemic, then fed them various foods to see which would make them recover most rapidly (Whipple was looking for treatments for anemia from bleeding, not pernicious anemia). Whipple discovered that ingesting large amounts of liver seemed to cure anemia from blood loss, and tried liver ingestion as a treatment for pernicious anemia, reporting improvement there also, in a paper in 1920. George Minot and William Murphy then set about to partly isolate the curative property in liver and showed in 1926 that it was contained in raw liver juice (in the process also showing that ironically it was the iron in liver tissue, not the soluble factor in liver juice, which cured the anemia from bleeding in dogs; thus the discovery of the liver juice factor as a treatment for pernicious anemia had been by coincidence). For the discovery of the cure of a previously fatal disease of unknown etiology, the three men shared the 1934 Nobel Prize in Medicine.

After Minot and Murphy's verification of Whipple's results in 1926, pernicious anemia victims ate or drank at least 1/2 a pound of raw liver, or drank raw liver juice, every day. This continued for several years, until a concentrate of liver juice became available. In 1928, chemist Edwin Cohn prepared a liver extract that was 50 to 100 times more potent than the natural food (liver). The extract could even be injected into muscle, which meant that patients no longer needed to eat large amounts of liver or juice. This also reduced the cost of treatment considerably.

The active ingredient in liver remained unknown until 1948, when it was isolated by two chemists, Karl A. Folkers of the United States and Alexander R. Todd of Great Britain. The substance was a cobalamin, which the discoverers named vitamin B_{12}. The new vitamin in liver juice was eventually completely purified and characterized in the 1950s, and other methods of producing it from bacteria were developed. It could be injected into muscle with even less irritation, making it possible to treat pernicious anemia with even more ease. Pernicious anemia was eventually treated with either vitamin B_{12} injections, or else large oral doses of vitamin B_{12}, typically between 1 and 4 mg (1000 to 4000 mcg) daily.

Notable cases

- Alexander Graham Bell - Scottish-Canadian scientist and inventor
- Annie Oakley
- Norman Warne - editor/publisher and fiancé of Beatrix Potter.
- Yoon Eun Hye - a South Korean actress

External links

- The Pernicious Anaemia Society [6], a UK-based charitable organization
- Parietal cell antibody [7]
- Antibody to GPC [8]
- [3]

Signs and Symptoms

Hypertension

Hypertension	
Classification and external resources	
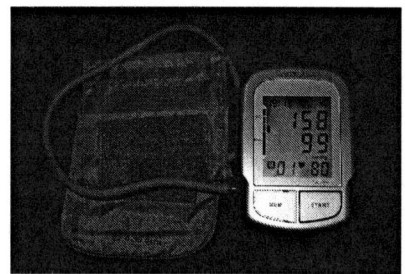Automated arm blood pressure meter showing arterial hypertension (shown a systolic blood pressure 158 mmHg, diastolic blood pressure 99 mmHg and heart rate of 80 beats per minute).	
ICD-10	I 10. [1],I 11. [2],I 12. [3], I 13. [4],I 15. [5]
ICD-9	401 [6]
OMIM	145500 [7]
DiseasesDB	6330 [8]
MedlinePlus	000468 [9]
eMedicine	med/1106 [10] ped/1097 [11] emerg/267 [12]
MeSH	D006973 [13]

Hypertension (HTN) or **high blood pressure** is a chronic medical condition in which the systemic arterial blood pressure is elevated. It is the opposite of hypotension. It is classified as either primary (essential) or secondary. About 90–95% of cases are termed "primary hypertension", which refers to high blood pressure for which no medical cause can be found. The remaining 5–10% of cases (Secondary hypertension) are caused by other conditions that affect the kidneys, arteries, heart, or endocrine system.

Persistent hypertension is one of the risk factors for stroke, myocardial infarction, heart failure and arterial aneurysm, and is a leading cause of chronic kidney failure. Moderate elevation of arterial blood pressure leads to shortened life expectancy. Dietary and lifestyle changes can improve blood pressure control and decrease the risk of associated health complications, although drug treatment may prove necessary in patients for whom lifestyle changes prove ineffective or insufficient.

Classification

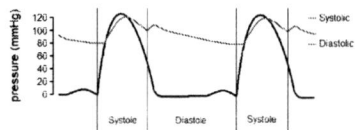

The variation in pressure in the left ventricle (blue line) and the aorta (red line) over two cardiac cycles ("heart beats"), showing the definitions of systolic and diastolic pressure

Classification	Systolic pressure		Diastolic pressure	
	mmHg	kPa	mmHg	kPa
Normal	90–119	12–15.9	60–79	8.0–10.5
Prehypertension	120–139	16.0–18.5	80–89	10.7–11.9
Stage 1	140–159	18.7–21.2	90–99	12.0–13.2
Stage 2	≥160	≥21.3	≥100	≥13.3
Isolated systolic hypertension	≥140	≥18.7	<90	<12.0
Source: American Heart Association (2003).				

Blood pressure is usually classified based on the systolic and diastolic blood pressures. Systolic blood pressure is the blood pressure in vessels during a heart beat. Diastolic blood pressure is the pressure between heartbeats. A systolic or the diastolic blood pressure measurement higher than the accepted normal values for the age of the individual is classified as prehypertension or hypertension.

Hypertension has several sub-classifications including, hypertension stage I, hypertension stage II, and isolated systolic hypertension. Isolated systolic hypertension refers to elevated systolic pressure with normal diastolic pressure and is common in the elderly. These classifications are made after averaging a patient's resting blood pressure readings taken on two or more office visits. Individuals older than 50 years are classified as having hypertension if their blood pressure is consistently at least 140 mmHg systolic or 90 mmHg diastolic. Patients with blood pressures higher than 130/80 mmHg with concomitant presence of diabetes mellitus or kidney disease require further treatment.

Hypertension is also classified as resistant if medications do not reduce blood pressure to normal levels.

Exercise hypertension is an excessively high elevation in blood pressure during exercise. The range considered normal for systolic values during exercise is between 200 and 230 mm Hg. Exercise hypertension may indicate that an individual is at risk for developing hypertension at rest.

Signs and symptoms

Mild to moderate essential hypertension is usually asymptomatic.

Accelerated hypertension

Accelerated hypertension is associated with headache, drowsiness, confusion, vision disorders, nausea, and vomiting symptoms which are collectively referred to as hypertensive encephalopathy.. Hypertensive encephalopathy is caused by severe small blood vessel congestion and brain swelling, which is reversible if blood pressure is lowered.

Children

Some signs and symptoms are especially important in newborns and infants such as failure to thrive, seizures, irritability, lack of energy, and difficulty breathing. In children, hypertension can cause headache, fatigue, blurred vision, nosebleeds, and facial paralysis.

Secondary hypertension

Some additional signs and symptoms suggest that the hypertension is caused by disorders in hormone regulation. Hypertension combined with obesity distributed on the trunk of the body, accumlated fat on the back of the neck ('buffalo hump'), wide purple marks on the abdomen (abdominal striae), or the recent on set of diabetes suggests that an individual has a hormone disorder known as Cushing's syndrome. Hypertension caused by other hormone disorders such as hyperthyroidism, hypothyroidism, or growth hormone excess will be accompanied by additional symptoms specific to these disorders. For example, hyperthyrodism can cause weight loss, tremors, heart rate abnormalities, reddening of the palms, and increased sweating. Signs and symptoms associated with growth hormone excess include coarsening of facial features, protrusion of the lower jaw, enlargement of the tongue, excessive hair growth, darkening of the skin color, and excessive sweating.[:499]. Other hormone disorders like hyperaldosteronism may cause less specific symptoms such as numbness, excessive urination, excessive sweating, electrolyte imbalances and dehydration, and elevated blood alkalinity. and also cause of mental pressure.

Pregnancy

Hypertension in pregnant women is known as pre-eclampsia. Pre-eclampsia can progress to a life-threatening condition called eclampsia, which is the development of protein in the urine, generalized swelling, and severe seizures. Other symptoms indicating that brain function is becoming impaired may precede these seizures such as nausea, vomiting, headaches, and vision loss.

Causes

Essential hypertension

Main article: Essential hypertension

Essential hypertension is the most prevalent hypertension type, affecting 90–95% of hypertensive patients. Although no direct cause has identified itself, there are many factors such as sedentary lifestyle, stress, visceral obesity, potassium deficiency (hypokalemia), obesity (more than 85% of cases occur in those with a body mass index greater than 25), salt (sodium) sensitivity, alcohol intake, and vitamin D deficiency that increase the risk of developing hypertension. Risk also increases with aging, some inherited genetic mutations, and having a family history of hypertension. An elevation of renin, a hormone secreted by the kidney, is another risk factor, as is sympathetic nervous system overactivity. Insulin resistance which is a component of syndrome X, or the metabolic syndrome is also thought to contribute to hypertension. Recent studies have implicated low birth weight as a risk factor for adult essential hypertension.

Secondary hypertension

Main article: Secondary hypertension

Secondary hypertension by definition results from an identifiable cause. This type is important to recognize since it's treated differently than essential hypertension, by treating the underlying cause of the elevated blood pressure. Hypertension results in the compromise or imbalance of the pathophysiological mechanisms, such as the hormone-regulating endocrine system, that regulate blood plasma volume and heart function. Many conditions cause hypertension, some are common and well recognized secondary causes such as Cushing's syndrome, which is a condition where the adrenal glands overproduce the hormone cortisol. In addition, hypertension is caused by other conditions that cause hormone changes such as hyperthyroidism, hypothyroidism (citation needed), and certain tumors of the adrenal medulla (e.g., pheochromocytoma). Other common causes of secondary hypertension include kidney disease, obesity/metabolic disorder, pre-eclampsia during pregnancy, the congenital defect known as coarctation of the aorta, and certain prescription and illegal drugs.

Pathophysiology

Main article: Pathophysiology of hypertension

Most of the mechanisms associated with secondary hypertension are generally fully understood. However, those associated with essential (primary) hypertension are far less understood. What is known is that cardiac output is raised early in the disease course, with total peripheral resistance (TPR)

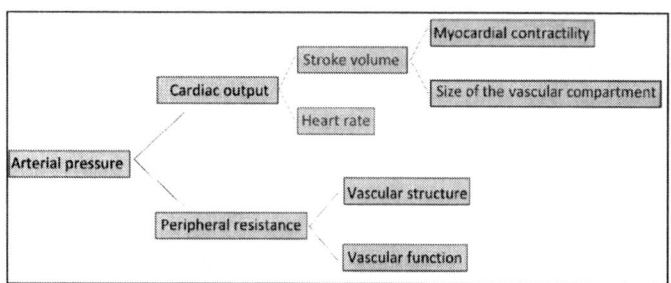

A diagram explaining factors affecting arterial pressure

normal; over time cardiac output drops to normal levels but TPR is increased. Three theories have been proposed to explain this:

- Inability of the kidneys to excrete sodium, resulting in natriuretic factors such as Atrial Natriuretic Factor being secreted to promote salt excretion with the side effect of raising total peripheral resistance.
- An overactive Renin-angiotensin system leads to vasoconstriction and retention of sodium and water. The increase in blood volume leads to hypertension.
- An overactive sympathetic nervous system, leading to increased stress responses.

It is also known that hypertension is highly heritable and polygenic (caused by more than one gene) and a few candidate genes have been postulated in the etiology of this condition.

Recently, work related to the association between essential hypertension and sustained endothelial damage has gained popularity among hypertension scientists. It remains unclear however whether endothelial changes precede the development of hypertension or whether such changes are mainly due to long standing elevated blood pressures.

Diagnosis

Hypertension is generally diagnosed on the basis of a persistently high blood pressure. Usually this requires three separate sphygmomanometer (see figure) measurements at least one week apart. Initial assessment of the hypertensive patient should include a complete history and physical examination. Exceptionally, if the elevation is extreme, or if symptoms of organ damage are present then the diagnosis may be given and treatment started immediately.

Once the diagnosis of hypertension has been made, physicians will attempt to identify the underlying cause based on risk factors and other symptoms, if present. Secondary hypertension is more common in preadolescent children, with most cases caused by renal disease. Primary or essential hypertension is more common in adolescents and has multiple risk factors, including obesity and a family history of hypertension. Laboratory tests can also be performed to identify possible causes of secondary hypertension, and determine if hypertension has caused damage to the heart, eyes, and kidneys. Additional tests for Diabetes and high cholesterol levels are also usually performed because they are additional risk factors for the development of heart disease require treatment. Tests typically performed are classified as follows:

System	Tests
Renal	Microscopic urinalysis, proteinuria, serum BUN (blood urea nitrogen) and/or creatinine
Endocrine	Serum sodium, potassium, calcium, TSH (thyroid-stimulating hormone).
Metabolic	Fasting blood glucose, total cholesterol, HDL and LDL cholesterol, triglycerides
Other	Hematocrit, electrocardiogram, and chest radiograph
Sources: *Harrison's principles of internal medicine others*	

Creatinine (renal function) testing is done to determine if kidney disease is present, which can be either the cause or result of hypertension. In addition, it provides a baseline measurement of kidney function that can be used to monitor for side-effects of certain antihypertensive drugs on kidney function. Additionally, testing of urine samples for protein is used as a secondary indicator of kidney disease. Glucose testing is done to determine if diabetes mellitus is present. Electrocardiogram (EKG/ECG) testing is done to check for evidence of the heart being under strain from high blood pressure. It may also show if there is thickening of the heart muscle (left ventricular hypertrophy) or has experienced a prior minor heart distubance such as a silent heart attack. A chest X-ray may be performed to look for signs of heart enlargement or damage to heart tissue.

Prevention

The degree to which hypertension can be prevented depends on a number of features including current blood pressure level, sodium/potassium balance, detection and omission of environmental toxins, changes in end/target organs (retina, kidney, heart, among others), risk factors for cardiovascular diseases and the age at diagnosis of prehypertension or at risk for hypertension. A prolonged assessment in which repeated measurements of blood pressure are taken provides the most accurate assessment of blood pressure levels. Following this, lifestyle changes are recommended to lower blood pressure, before the initiation of prescription drug therapy. The process of managing prehypertension according the guidelines of the British Hypertension Society suggest the following lifestyle changes:

- Weight reduction and regular aerobic exercise (e.g., walking): Regular exercise improves blood flow and helps to reduce the resting heart rate and blood pressure.
- Reducing dietary sugar.

- Reducing sodium (salt) in the diet: This step decreases blood pressure in about 33% of people (see above). Many people use a salt substitute to reduce their salt intake.
- Additional dietary changes beneficial to reducing blood pressure include the DASH diet (**d**ietary **a**pproaches to **s**top **h**ypertension) which is rich in fruits and vegetables and low-fat or fat-free dairy products. This diet has been shown to be effective based on research sponsored by the National Heart, Lung, and Blood Institute. In addition, an increase in dietary potassium, which offsets the effect of sodium has been shown to be highly effective in reducing blood pressure.
- Discontinuing tobacco use and alcohol consumption has been shown to lower blood pressure. The exact mechanisms are not fully understood, but blood pressure (especially systolic) always transiently increases following alcohol or nicotine consumption. Abstaining from cigarette smoking reduces the risk of stroke and heart attack which are associated with hypertension.
- Reducing stress, for example with relaxation therapy, such as meditation and other mindbody relaxation techniques, by reducing environmental stress such as high sound levels and over-illumination can also lower blood pressure. Jacobson's Progressive Muscle Relaxation and biofeedback are also beneficial, such as device-guided paced breathing, although meta-analysis suggests it is not effective unless combined with other relaxation techniques.

Treatment

Lifestyle modifications

The first line of treatment for hypertension is the same as the recommended preventative lifestyle changes such as the dietary changes, physical exercise, and weight loss, which have all been shown to significantly reduce blood pressure in people with hypertension. If hypertension is high enough to justify immediate use of medications, lifestyle changes are still recommended in conjunction with medication. Drug prescription should take into account the patient's absolute cardiovascular risk (including risk of myocardial infarction and stroke) as well as blood pressure readings, in order to gain a more accurate picture of the patient's cardiovascular profile. Different programs aimed to reduce psychological stress such as biofeedback, relaxation or meditation are advertised to reduce hypertension. However, in general claims of efficacy are not supported by scientific studies, which have been in general of low quality.

Regarding dietary changes, a low sodium diet is beneficial; A Cochrane review published in 2008 concluded that a long term (more than 4 weeks) low sodium diet in Caucasians has a useful effect to reduce blood pressure, both in people with hypertension and in people with normal blood pressure. Also, the DASH diet (Dietary Approaches to Stop Hypertension) is a diet promoted by the National Heart, Lung, and Blood Institute (part of the NIH, a United States government organization) to control hypertension. A major feature of the plan is limiting intake of sodium, and it also generally encourages the consumption of nuts, whole grains, fish, poultry, fruits and vegetables while lowering the consumption of red meats, sweets, and sugar. It is also "rich in potassium, magnesium, and calcium, as well as protein".

Medications

Main article: Antihypertensive drug

Several classes of medications, collectively referred to as antihypertensive drugs, are currently available for treating hypertension. Agents within a particular class generally share a similar pharmacologic mechanism of action, and in many cases have an affinity for similar cellular receptors. An exception to this rule is the diuretics, which are grouped together for the sake of simplicity but actually exert their effects by a number of different mechanisms.

Reduction of the blood pressure by 5 mmHg can decrease the risk of stroke by 34%, of ischaemic heart disease by 21%, and reduce the likelihood of dementia, heart failure, and mortality from cardiovascular disease. The aim of treatment should be reduce blood pressure to <140/90 mmHg for most individuals, and lower for individuals with diabetes or kidney disease (some medical professionals recommend keeping levels below 120/80 mmHg). Comorbidity also plays a role in determining target blood pressure, with lower BP targets applying to patients with end-organ damage or proteinuria.

Often multiple drugs are combined to achieve the goal blood pressure. Commonly used prescription drugs include:

- ACE inhibitors (e.g., captopril)
- Alpha blockers (e.g., prazosin)
- Angiotensin II receptor antagonists (e.g., losartan)
- Beta blockers (e.g., propranolol)
- Calcium channel blockers (e.g., verapamil)
- Diuretics (e.g. hydrochlorothiazide)
- Direct renin inhibitors (e.g., aliskiren)

Some examples of common combined prescription drug treatments include:

- A fixed combination of an ACE inhibitor and a calcium channel blocker. One example of this is the combination of perindopril and amlodipine, the efficacy of which has been demonstrated in individuals with glucose intolerance or metabolic syndrome.
- A fixed combination of an ACE inhibitor and a calcium channel blocker.
- A fixed combination of a diuretic and an ARB.

Resistant

Guidelines for treating resistant hypertension have been published in the UK and US.

Complications

Main article: Complications of hypertension

Hypertension is the most important risk factor for death in industrialized countries. It increases hardening of the arteries thus predisposes individuals to heart disease, peripheral vascular disease, and strokes. Types of heart disease that may occur include: myocardial infarction, heart failure, and left ventricular hypertrophy Other complications include:

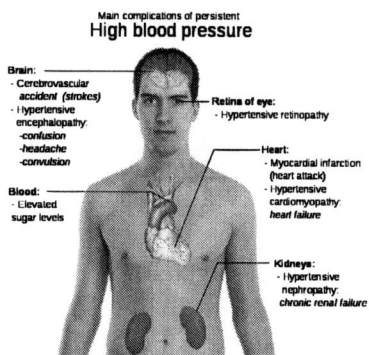

Diagram illustrating the main complications of persistent high blood pressure.

* Hypertensive retinopathy
* Hypertensive nephropathy
* If blood pressure is very high hypertensive encephalopathy may result.

Epidemiology

In the year 2000 it is estimated that nearly one billion people or ~26% of the adult population have hypertension worldwide. It was common in both developed (333 million) and undeveloped (639 million) countries. However rates vary markedly in different regions with rates as low as 3.4% (men) and 6.8% (women) in rural India and as high as 68.9% (men) and 72.5% (women) in Poland.

In 1995 it is estimated that 43 million people in the United States had hypertension or were taking antihypertensive medication, almost 24% of the adult population. The prevalence of hypertension in the United States is increasing and reached 29% in 2004. It is more common in blacks and less in whites and Mexican Americans, rates increase with age, and is greater in the southeastern United States. Hypertension is more prevalent in men (though menopause tends to decrease this difference) and those of low socioeconomic status.

Over 90–95% of adult hypertension is essential hypertension. The most common cause of secondary hypertension is primary aldosteronism. The incidence of exercise hypertension is reported to range from 1–10%.

Pediatrics

The prevalence of high blood pressure in the young is increasing. Most childhood hypertension, particularly in preadolescents, is secondary to an underlying disorder. Kidney disease is the most common (60–70%) cause of hypertension in children. Adolescents usually have primary or essential hypertension, which accounts for 85–95% of cases.

History

Some cite the writings of Sushruta in the 6th century BC as being the first mention of symptoms like those of hypertension. Others propose even earlier descriptions dating as far as 2600 years before Christ. Main treatment for what was called the "hard pulse disease" consisted in reducing the quantity of blood in a subject by the sectioning of veins or the application of leeches. Well known individuals such as The Yellow Emperor of China, Cornelius Celsus, Galen, and Hipocrates advocated such treatments.

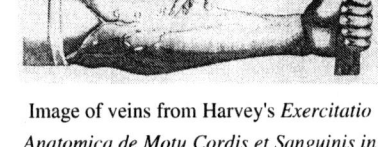

Image of veins from Harvey's *Exercitatio Anatomica de Motu Cordis et Sanguinis in Animalibus*

Our modern understanding of hypertension began with the work of physician William Harvey (1578–1657), who was the first to describe correctly the systemic circulation of blood being pumped around the body by the heart in his book "*De motu cordis*". The basis for measuring blood pressure were established by Stephen Hales in 1733. Initial descriptions of hypertension as a disease came among others from Thomas Young in 1808 and specially Richard Bright in 1836. The first ever elevated blood pressure in a patient without kidney disease was reported by Frederick Mahomed (1849–1884). It was not until 1904 that sodium restriction was advocated while a rice diet was popularized around 1940.

Studies in the 1920s demonstrated the public health impact of untreated high blood pressure; treatment options were limited at the time, and deaths from malignant hypertension and its complications were common. A prominent victim of severe hypertension leading to cerebral hemorrhage was Franklin D. Roosevelt (1882–1945). The Framingham Heart Study added to the epidemiological understanding of hypertension and its relationship with coronary artery disease. The National Institutes of Health also sponsored other population studies, which additionally showed that African Americans had a higher burden of hypertension and its complications. Before pharmacological treatment for hypertension became possible, three treatment modalities were used, all with numerous side-effects: strict sodium restriction, sympathectomy (surgical ablation of parts of the sympathetic nervous system), and pyrogen therapy (injection of substances that caused a fever, indirectly reducing blood pressure).

The first chemical for hypertension, sodium thiocyanate, was used in 1900 but had many side effects and was unpopular. Several other agents were developed after the Second World War, the most popular and reasonably effective of which were tetramethylammonium chloride and its derivative hexamethonium, hydralazine and reserpine (derived from the medicinal plant *Rauwolfia serpentina*). A randomized controlled trial sponsored by the Veterans Administration using these drugs had to be stopped early because those not receiving treatment were developing more complications and it was deemed unethical to withhold treatment from them. These studies prompted public health campaigns to increase public awareness of hypertension and the advice to get blood pressure measured and treated. These measures appear to have contributed at least in part of the observed 50% fall in stroke and ischemic heart disease beween 1972 and 1994.

A major breakthrough was achieved with the discovery of the first well-tolerated orally available agents. The first was chlorothiazide, the first thiazide and developed from the antibiotic sulfanilamide, which became available in 1958; it increased salt excretion while preventing fluid accumulation. In 1975, the Lasker Special Public Health Award was awarded to the team that developed chlorothiazide. The British physician James W. Black developed beta blockers in the early 1960s; these were initially used for angina, but turned out to lower blood pressure. Black received the 1976 Lasker Award and in 1988 the Nobel Prize in Physiology or Medicine for his discovery. The next class of antihypertensives to be discovered was that of the calcium channel blockers. The first member was verapamil, a derivative of papaverine that was initially thought to be a beta blocker and used for angina, but then turned out to have a different mode of action and was shown to lower blood pressure. ACE inhibitors were developed through rational drug design; the renin-angiotensin system was known to play an important role in blood pressure regulation, and snake venom from *Bothrops jararaca* could lower blood pressure through inhibition of ACE. In 1977 captopril, an orally active agent, was described; this led to the development of a number of other ACE inhibitors.

Society and culture

Economics

The National Heart, Lung, and Blood Institute (NHLBI) estimated in 2002 that hypertension cost the United States $47.2 billion.

High blood pressure is the most common chronic medical problem prompting visits to primary health care providers, yet it is estimated that only 34% of the 50 million American adults with hypertension have their blood pressure controlled to a level of <140/90 mm Hg [citation needed]. Thus, about two thirds of Americans with hypertension are at increased risk for heart disease. The medical, economic, and human costs of untreated and inadequately controlled high blood pressure are enormous. Adequate management of hypertension can be hampered by inadequacies in the diagnosis, treatment, and/or control of high blood pressure. Health care providers face many obstacles to achieving blood pressure control from their patients, including resistance to taking multiple medications to reach blood pressure goals. Patients also face the challenges of adhering to medicine schedules and making lifestyle changes.

Nonetheless, the achievement of blood pressure goals is possible, and most importantly, lowering blood pressure significantly reduces the risk of death due to heart disease, the development of other debilitating conditions, and the cost associated with advanced medical care.,

Awareness

The World Health Organization attributes hypertension, or high blood pressure, as the leading cause of cardiovascular mortality. The World Hypertension League (WHL), an umbrella organization of 85 national hypertension societies and leagues, recognized that more than 50% of the hypertensive population worldwide are unaware of their condition. To address this problem, the WHL initiated a global awareness campaign on hypertension in 2005 and dedicated May 17 of each year as World Hypertension Day (WHD). Over the past three years, more national societies have been engaging in WHD and have been innovative in

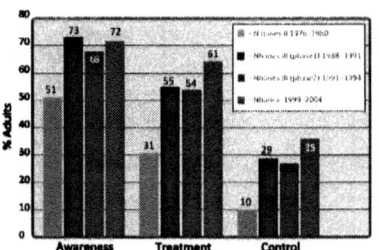

Graph showing, prevalence of awareness, treatment and control of hypertension compared between the four studies of NHANES

their activities to get the message to the public. In 2007, there was record participation from 47 member countries of the WHL. During the week of WHD, all these countries – in partnership with their local governments, professional societies, nongovernmental organizations and private industries – promoted hypertension awareness among the public through several media and public rallies. Using mass media such as Internet and television, the message reached more than 250 million people. As the momentum picks up year after year, the WHL is confident that almost all the estimated 1.5 billion people affected by elevated blood pressure can be reached.

Further reading

- Oke DA, Bandele EO (September 2004). "Misconceptions of hypertension" [14]. *Journal of the National Medical Association* **96** (9): 1221–4. PMID 15481752 [15].
- The American Journal of Hypertension [16]

External links

- The Framingham Heart Study [17]
- Video showing how to measure blood pressure [18]
- Hypertension [19] at the Open Directory Project
- High Blood Pressure [20] from the Heart and Stroke Foundation of Canada
- High Blood Pressure [21] from MedlinePlus
- A guide to lowering high blood pressure [22] from the National Heart, Lung, and Blood Institute

- High Blood Pressure [23] (from the American Heart Association)
- Pulmonary Hypertension [24] from Cleveland Clinic Online Medical Reference

Hypotension

Hypotension	
Classification and external resources	
ICD-10	I 95. [1]
ICD-9	458 [2]
DiseasesDB	6539 [3]
MedlinePlus	007278 [4]
MeSH	D007022 [5]

In physiology and medicine, **hypotension** is abnormally low blood pressure. This is best understood as a physiologic state, rather than a disease. It is often associated with shock, though not necessarily indicative of it. Hypotension is the opposite of hypertension, which is high blood pressure. Blood pressure is the force of blood pushing against the walls of the arteries as the heart pumps out blood. If it is lower than normal then it is called **low blood pressure** or hypotension. There is no specific number at which day-to-day blood pressure is considered too low, as long as no symptoms of trouble are present

Signs and symptoms

The cardinal symptom of hypotension is lightheadedness or dizziness. If the blood pressure is sufficiently low, fainting and often seizures will occur.

Low blood pressure is sometimes associated with certain symptoms, many of which are related to causes rather than effects of hypotension:

- Chest pain
- Shortness of breath
- Irregular heartbeat
- Fever higher than 101 °F (38.3 °C)
- Headache
- Stiff neck
- Severe upper back pain

- Cough with phlegm
- Prolonged diarrhea or vomiting
- Dysphagia
- Dysuria
- Foul-smelling urine
- Adverse effect of medications
- Acute, life-threatening allergic reaction
- Seizures
- Loss of consciousness
- Profound fatigue
- Temporary blurring or loss of vision
- In some cases loss of hair
- Ehlers-Danlos Syndrome

Cause

Low blood pressure causes can be due to hormonal changes, widening of blood vessels, medicine side effects, anemia, heart & endocrine problems.

Reduced blood volume, called hypovolemia, is the most common mechanism producing hypotension. This can result from hemorrhage, or blood loss; insufficient fluid intake, as in starvation; or excessive fluid losses from diarrhea or vomiting. Hypovolemia is often induced by excessive use of diuretics. Other medications can produce hypotension by different mechanisms.

Decreased cardiac output despite normal blood volume, due to severe congestive heart failure, large myocardial infarction, or bradycardia, often produces hypotension and can rapidly progress to cardiogenic shock. Arrhythmias often result in hypotension by this mechanism. Beta blockers can cause hypotension both by slowing the heart rate and by decreasing the pumping ability of the heart muscle. Varieties of meditation and/or other mental-physiological disciplines can create temporary hypotension effects, as well, and should not be considered unusual.

Excessive vasodilation, or insufficient constriction of the resistance blood vessels (mostly arterioles), causes hypotension. This can be due to decreased sympathetic nervous system output or to increased parasympathetic activity occurring as a consequence of injury to the brain or spinal cord or of dysautonomia, an intrinsic abnormality in autonomic system functioning. Excessive vasodilation can also result from sepsis, acidosis, or medications, such as nitrate preparations, calcium channel blockers, angiotensin II receptor blockers ACE inhibitors. Many anesthetic agents and techniques, including spinal anesthesia and most inhalational agents, produce significant vasodilation.

Pathophysiology

Blood pressure is continuously regulated by the autonomic nervous system, using an elaborate network of receptors, nerves, and hormones to balance the effects of the sympathetic nervous system, which tends to raise blood pressure, and the parasympathetic nervous system, which lowers it. The vast and rapid compensation abilities of the autonomic nervous system allow normal individuals to maintain an acceptable blood pressure over a wide range of activities and in many disease states.

Syndromes

Orthostatic hypotension, also called "postural hypotension", is a common form of low blood pressure. It occurs after a change in body position, typically when a person stands up from either a seated or lying position. It is usually transient and represents a delay in the normal compensatory ability of the autonomic nervous system. It is commonly seen in hypovolemia and as a result of various medications. In addition to blood pressure-lowering medications, many psychiatric medications, in particular antidepressants, can have this side effect. Simple blood pressure and heart rate measurements while lying, seated, and standing (with a two-minute delay in between each position change) can confirm the presence of orthostatic hypotension. Orthostatic hypotension is indicated if there is a drop in 20 mmHg of systolic pressure (and a 10 mmHg drop in diastolic pressure in some facilities) and a 20 bpm increase in heart rate.

Neurocardiogenic syncope is a form of dysautonomia characterized by an inappropriate drop in blood pressure while in the upright position. Neurocardiogenic syncope is related to vasovagal syncope in that both occur as a result of increased activity of the vagus nerve, the mainstay of the parasympathetic nervous system.

Another, but rarer form, is postprandial hypotension, which occurs 30–75 minutes after eating substantial meals. When a great deal of blood is diverted to the intestines (a kind of "splanchnic blood pooling") to facilitate digestion and absorption, the body must increase cardiac output and peripheral vasoconstriction in order to maintain enough blood pressure to perfuse vital organs, such as the brain. It is believed that postprandial hypotension is caused by the autonomic nervous system not compensating appropriately, because of aging or a specific disorder.

Diagnosis

For most adults, the healthiest blood pressure is at or below 115/75 mmHg. A small drop in blood pressure, even as little as 20 mmHg, can result in transient hypotension.

Evaluation of neurocardiogenic syncope is done with a tilt table test.

Treatment

The treatment for hypotension depends on its cause. Chronic hypotension rarely exists as more than a symptom. Asymptomatic hypotension in healthy people usually does not require treatment. Adding electrolytes to a diet can relieve symptoms of mild hypotension. In mild cases, where the patient is still responsive, laying the person in dorsal decubitus (lying on the back) position and lifting the legs will increase venous return, thus making more blood available to critical organs at the chest and head. The Trendelenburg position, though used historically, is no longer recommended.

The treatment of hypotensive shock always follows the first four following steps. Outcomes, in terms of mortality, are directly linked to the speed in which hypotension is corrected. In parentheses are the still debated methods for achieving, and benchmarks for evaluating, progress in correcting hypotension. A study on *Early Goal Directed Therapy* provided the delineation of these general principles. However, since it focuses on hypotension due to infection, it is not applicable to all forms of severe hypotension.

1. Volume resuscitation (usually with crystalloid)
2. Blood pressure support (with norepinephrine or equivalent)
3. Ensure adequate tissue perfusion (maintain SvO2 >70 with use of blood or dobutamine)
4. Address the underlying problem (i.e. antibiotic for infection, stent or CABG for infarction, steroids for adrenal insufficiency, etc...)

Medium-term (and less well-demonstrated) treatments of hypotension include:

- Blood sugar control (80-150 by one study)
- Early nutrition (by mouth or by tube to prevent ileus)
- Steroid support

See also

- Hypotensive transfusion reaction

External links

- Understanding Low Blood Pressure - the Basics [6] WebMD

Fatigue (medical)

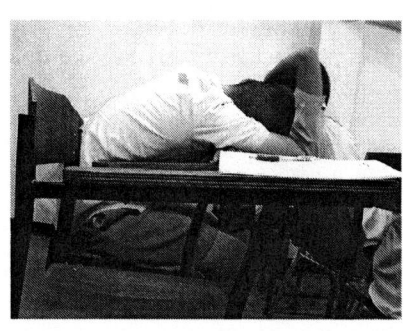

Occupations that require an individual to work long hours and stay up overnight can lead to fatigue.

ICD-10	R 53. [1]
ICD-9	780.7 [2]
DiseasesDB	30079 [3]
MedlinePlus	003088 [4]
MeSH	D005221 [5]

Fatigue (also called **exhaustion, lethargy, languidness, languor, lassitude,** and **listlessness**) is a state of awareness describing a range of afflictions, usually associated with physical and/or mental weakness, though varying from a general state of lethargy to a specific work-induced burning sensation within one's muscles. Physical fatigue is the inability to continue functioning at the level of one's normal abilities. It is ubiquitous in everyday life, but usually becomes particularly noticeable during heavy exercise. Mental fatigue, on the other hand, rather manifests in somnolence (sleepiness).

Fatigue is considered a symptom, as opposed to a medical sign, because it is reported by the patient instead of being observed by others. Fatigue and 'feelings of fatigue' are often confused.

Types

Physical fatigue

Main article: Muscle weakness

Physical fatigue or muscle weakness (or "lack of strength") is a direct term for the inability to exert force with one's muscles to the degree that would be expected given the individual's general physical fitness.

A test of strength is often used during a diagnosis of a muscular disorder before the etiology can be identified. Such etiology depends on the type of muscle weakness, which can be true or perceived as well as central or peripheral. True weakness is substantial, while perceived rather is a sensation of having to put more effort to do the same task. On the other hand, central muscle weakness is an overall exhaustion of the whole body, while peripheral weakness is an exhaustion of individual muscles.

Mental fatigue

See also: Somnolence

In addition to physical, fatigue also includes mental fatigue, not necessarily including any muscle fatigue. Such a mental fatigue, in turn, can manifest itself both as somnolence (decreased wakefulness) or just as a general decrease of attention, not necessarily including sleepiness. It may also be described as a more or less decreased level of consciousness. In any case, this can be dangerous when performing tasks that require constant concentration, such as driving a vehicle. For instance, a person who is sufficiently somnolent may experience microsleeps. However, objective cognitive testing should be done to differentiate the neurocognitive deficits of brain disease from those attributable to tiredness.

Differential diagnosis

The majority of people who have fatigue do not have an underlying cause discovered after a year with the condition. In those who do have a possible diagnosis musculoskeletal (19.4%) and psychological problems (16.5%) are the most common. Definitive physical conditions were only found in 8.2%.

Fatigue is typically the result of working, mental stress, overstimulation and understimulation, jet lag or active recreation, depression, and also boredom, disease and lack of sleep. It may also have chemical causes, such as poisoning or mineral or vitamin deficiencies. Massive blood loss frequently results in fatigue. Fatigue is different from drowsiness, where a patient feels that sleep is required. Fatigue is a normal response to physical exertion or stress, but can also be a sign of a physical disorder.

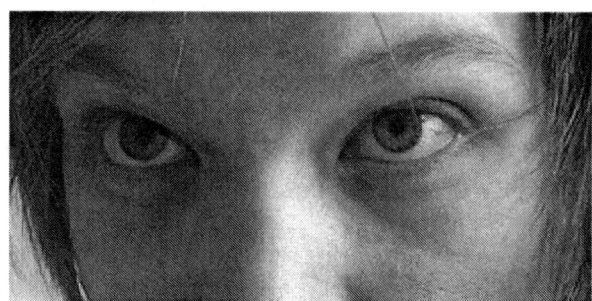

Minor dark circles, in addition to a hint of eye bags, a combination mainly suggestive of minor sleep deprivation.

The sense of fatigue is believed to originate in the reticular activating system of the lower brain. Musculoskeletal structures may have co-evolved with appropriate brain structures so that the complete unit functions together in a constructive and adaptive fashion. The entire systems of muscles, joints, and proprioceptive and kinesthetic functions plus parts of the brain evolve and function together in a unitary way.

Temporary fatigue is likely to be a minor illness like the common cold as one part of the sickness behavior response that happens when the immune system fights an infection. Chronic fatigue, on the other hand, meaning of six months or more duration, is a symptom of a large number of different diseases or conditions. Some major categories of diseases that feature fatigue include:

- Autoimmune diseases such as celiac disease, multiple sclerosis, and spondyloarthropathy
- Blood disorders such as anemia and hemochromatosis
- Cancer
- Chronic fatigue syndrome (CFS)
- Depression and other mental disorders that feature depressed mood
- Eating disorders, which can produce fatigue due to inadequate nutrition
- Endocrine disease like diabetes mellitus and hypothyroidism
- Fibromyalgia
- Heart disease
- Infectious diseases such as infectious mononucleosis and influenza
- Leukemia or lymphoma

- Neurological disorders such as Parkinson's disease and post-concussion syndrome
- Physical trauma and other pain-causing conditions, such as arthritis
- Sleep deprivation or sleep disorders
- Uremia
- Hepatic failure

Medications

- Certain medications, e.g. lithium salts, ciprofloxacin
- Beta blocker medication causes fatigue, especially after exertion, inducing exercise intolerance.
- Many cancer treatments cause fatigue, particularly chemotherapy and radiotherapy

Diagnostics approach

After deciding to see a doctor for guidance and treatment against fatigue, the physician will look at a person's medical history along with the evaluation of the fatigue itself. When evaluating sleep, questions will be asked regarding the quality of sleep, emotional state of the person, sleep pattern, and stress level. Questions about a person's diet, exercise level, and the symptoms that they are experiencing will also be asked. The quality of sleep a person is receiving is important. Certain points like if there is a pattern of fatigue consistent with the same time of the day or if it progressively worsens throughout the day are looked at. It is important that a patient take note of specific areas of sleep and fatigue before the visit so that they have answers to the right questions. The amount of sleep, the hours that are set aside for sleep, and the number of times that a person awakes during the night are important. Other tests that might be ordered by the physician include blood tests to check for infection or anemia, urinalysis to look for signs of liver disease or diabetes, and tests to monitor the function of the thyroid. A common exam that monitors the levels of seven common substances found circulating in the blood is also used. It consists of the four electrolytes:sodium, potassium, chloride, and bicarbonate, along with two waste products of metabolism (cleared by normally functioning kidneys) which are BUN and creatinine, and lastly, the source of energy for your body's cells, glucose. Specific tests will be run to check for HIV and female patients will also be required to receive a pregnancy test.

See also

Other fatigue-related articles

- Fatigue (safety)
- Sleep deprived driving
- Combat stress reaction (Battle fatigue)
- Cancer-related fatigue

Other medical symptoms and conditions

- Malaise
- Asthenia
- Paresis
- Debility
- Muscle fatigue
- Eye circles

References

- Gandevia SC (1992). "Some central and peripheral factors affecting human motoneuronal output in neuromuscular fatigue". *Sports medicine (Auckland, N.Z.)* **13** (2): 93–8. doi:10.2165/00007256-199213020-00004 [6]. PMID 1561512 [7].
- Hagberg M (1981). "Muscular endurance and surface electromyogram in isometric and dynamic exercise". *Journal of applied physiology: respiratory, environmental and exercise physiology* **51** (1): 1–7. PMID 7263402 [8].
- Hawley JA, Reilly T (1997). "Fatigue revisited". *Journal of sports sciences* **15** (3): 245–6. doi:10.1080/026404197367245 [9]. PMID 9232549 [10].
- Edelman, Gerald Maurice (1989). *The remembered present: a biological theory of consciousness.* New York: Basic Books. ISBN 0-465-06910-X.
- Kelso, J. A. Scott (1995). *Dynamic patterns: the self-organization of brain and behavior.* Cambridge, Mass: MIT Press. ISBN 0-262-61131-7.

External links

- Fatigue — Information for Patients [11], U.S. National Cancer Institute
- Tiredness [12] — Information leaflet from mental health charity The Royal College of Psychiatrists

Tachycardia

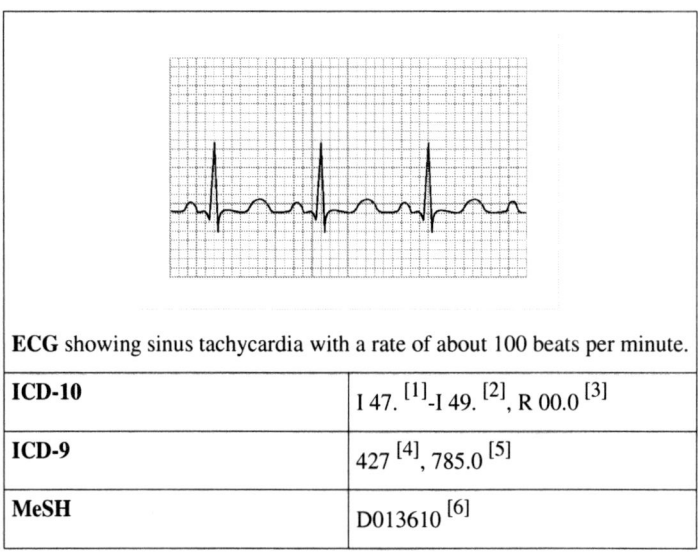

ECG showing sinus tachycardia with a rate of about 100 beats per minute.

ICD-10	I 47. [1]-I 49. [2], R 00.0 [3]
ICD-9	427 [4], 785.0 [5]
MeSH	D013610 [6]

Tachycardia comes from the Greek words **tachys** (*rapid* or *accelerated*) and *kardia* (*of the heart*). Tachycardia typically refers to a heart rate that exceeds the normal range for a resting heartrate (heartrate in an inactive or sleeping individual). It can be very dangerous depending on how hard the heart is working and the activity.

Definition

The upper threshold of a normal human heart rate is usually based upon age:

- 1–2 days: >159 beats per minute (bpm)
- 3–6 days: >166 bpm
- 1–3 weeks: >182 bpm
- 1–2 months: >179 bpm
- 3–5 months: >186 bpm
- 6–11 months: >169 bpm
- 1–2 years: >151 bpm
- 3–4 years: >137 bpm
- 5–7 years: >133 bpm
- 8–11 years: >130 bpm
- 12–15 years: >119 bpm
- >15 years – adult: >100 bpm

When the heart beats rapidly, the heart pumps less efficiently and provides less blood flow to the rest of the body, including the heart itself. The increased heart rate also leads to increased work and oxygen demand for the heart (myocardium), which can lead to rate related Ischemia thus perhaps causing a heart attack (myocardial infarction) if it persists. This occurs because the decreased flow of necessary oxygen to the heart causes myocardial cells to begin to die off. Acutely, this leads to angina; and chronically to ischemic heart disease.

Differential diagnosis

An electrocardiogram (ECG) can help distinguish between the various types of tachycardias, generally distinguished by their site of pacemaker origin:

12 lead electrocardiogram showing a run of ventricular tachycardia (VT)

- Sinus tachycardia, which originates from the sino-atrial (SA) node, near the base of the superior vena cava.
- Ventricular tachycardia, any tachycardia which originates in the ventricles.
- Supraventricular tachycardia (SVT), which is a tachycardia paced from the atria or the AV node. SVT rhythms include:

  - Atrial fibrillation
  - AV nodal reentrant tachycardia (AVNRT)
  - AV reentrant tachycardia (AVRT)
  - Junctional tachycardia

Tachycardias may be classified as either **narrow complex tachycardias** (supraventricular tachycardias) or **wide complex tachycardias**. "Narrow" and "wide" refer to the width of the QRS complex on the ECG. Narrow complex tachycardias tend to originate in the atria, while wide complex tachycardias tend to originate in the ventricles. Tachycardias can be further classified as either regular or irregular.

Sinus tachycardia

Main article: Sinus tachycardia

Ventricular tachycardia

Main article: Ventricular tachycardia

Ventricular tachycardia (VT or V-tach) is a potentially life-threatening cardiac arrhythmia that originates in the ventricles. It is usually a regular, wide complex tachycardia with a rate between 120 and 250 beats per minute. Ventricular tachycardia has the potential of degrading to the more serious ventricular fibrillation. Ventricular tachycardia is a common, and often lethal, complication of a myocardial infarction (heart attack).

Exercise-induced ventricular tachycardia is a phenomenon related to sudden deaths, especially in patients with severe heart disease (ischemia, acquired valvular heart and congenital heart disease) accompanied with left ventricular dysfunction. A case of a death from exercise-induced VT was the death on a basketball court of Hank Gathers, the Loyola Marymount basketball star, in March 1990.

Both of these rhythms normally last for only a few seconds to minutes *(paroxysmal tachycardia)*, but if VT persists it is extremely dangerous, often leading to ventricular fibrillation.

Supraventricular tachycardia

This is a type tachycardia that originates from above the ventricles, such as the atria. It is sometimes known as paroxysmal atrial tachycardia (PAT). Several types of supraventricular tachycardia are known to exist.

Main article: Supraventricular tachycardia

Atrial fibrillation

Atrial fibrillation is one of the most common cardiac arrhythmias. It is generally an irregular, narrow complex rhythm. However, it may show wide QRS complexes on the ECG if a bundle branch block is present. At high rates, the QRS complex may also become wide due to the Ashman phenomenon. It may be difficult to determine the rhythm's regularity when the rate exceeds 150 beats per minute. Depending on the patient's health and other variables such as medications taken for rate control, atrial fibrillation may cause heart rates that span from 50 to 250 beats per minute (or even higher if an accessory pathway is present). However, new onset atrial fibrillation tends to present with rates between 100 and 150 beats per minute.

AV nodal reentrant tachycardia (AVNRT)

AV nodal reentrant tachycardia is the most common reentrant tachycardia. It is a regular narrow complex tachycardia that usually responds well to the Valsalva maneuver or the drug adenosine. However, unstable patients sometimes require synchronized cardioversion. Definitive care may include catheter ablation.

AV reentrant tachycardia

AV reentrant tachycardia (AVRT) requires an accessory pathway for its maintenance. AVRT may involve orthodromic conduction (where the impulse travels down the AV node to the ventricles and back up to the atria through the accessory pathway) or antidromic conduction (which the impulse travels down the accessory pathway and back up to the atria through the AV node). Orthodromic conduction usually results in a narrow complex tachycardia, and antidromic conduction usually results in a wide complex tachycardia that often mimics ventricular tachycardia. Most antiarrhythmics are contraindicated in the emergency treatment of AVRT, because they may paradoxically increase conduction across the accessory pathway.

Junctional tachycardia

Junctional tachycardia is an automatic tachycardia originating in the AV junction. It tends to be a regular, narrow complex tachycardia and may be a sign of digitalis toxicity.

Hemodynamic responses

The body has several feedback mechanisms to maintain adequate blood flow and blood pressure. If blood pressure decreases, the heart beats faster in an attempt to raise it. This is called reflex tachycardia. This can happen in response to a decrease in blood volume (through dehydration or bleeding), or an unexpected change in blood flow. The most common cause of the latter is orthostatic hypotension (also called postural hypotension). Fever, hyperventilation and severe infections can also cause tachycardia, primarily due to increase in metabolic demands.

Autonomic and endocrine

An increase in sympathetic nervous system stimulation causes the heart rate to increase, both by the direct action of sympathetic nerve fibers on the heart and by causing the endocrine system to release hormones such as epinephrine (adrenaline), which have a similar effect. Increased sympathetic stimulation is usually due to physical or psychological stress. This is the basis for the so-called "Fight or Flight" response, but such stimulation can also be induced by stimulants such as ephedrine, amphetamines or cocaine. Certain endocrine disorders such as pheochromocytoma can also cause epinephrine release and can result in tachycardia independent nervous system stimulation. Hyperthyroidism can also cause tachycardia.

Management

The management of tachycardia depends on the underlying cause.

If it is due to an underlying cardiac conduction abnormality chemical conversion (with antiarrhythmics), electrical conversion (giving external shocks to convert the heart to a normal rhythm) or use of drugs to simply control heart rate may be used.

If the tachycardia originates from the sinus node (sinus tachycardia), treatment of the underlying cause of sinus tachycardia is usually sufficient. On the other hand, if the tachycardia is of a potentially lethal origin (i.e.: ventricular tachycardia) treatment with anti arrhythmic agents or with electrical cardioversion may be required. Below is a brief discussion of some of the main tachyarrhythmias and their treatments.

The electrocardiac management of atrial fibrillation and atrial flutter is either through medications or electrical cardioversion. Pharmacologic management of these arrhythmias typically involves diltiazem or verapamil as well as beta-blocking agents such as atenolol. The decision to use electrical cardioversion depends heavily on the hemodynamic stability of the presenting patient; in general those patients who are unable to sustain their systemic functions are electrically converted although conversion to a normal sinus rhythm can be performed with amiodarone. An interesting type of atrial fibrillation which must be carefully managed is when it appears in combination with Wolff-Parkinson-White syndrome. In this case, calcium channel blockers, beta-blockers and digoxin must be avoided to prevent precipitation of ventricular tachycardia. Here, procainamide or quinidine are often used. Of note: patients who have been in atrial fibrillation for more than 48 hours should not be converted to normal sinus rhythm unless they have been anti-coagulated to an INR of 2-3 for at least 4 weeks. This is to help prevent blood clots embolizing from the heart chambers to the rest of the body where they can cause adverse events like a stroke.

In the case of narrow complex tachycardias (junctional, atrial or paroxysmal), the treatment in general is to first give the patient adenosine (to slow conduction through the AV node) and then perform Valsalva maneuvers to slow the rhythm. If this does not convert the patient, amiodarone, calcium channel blockers or beta-blockers are commonly employed to stabilize the patient. Again as in atrial fibrillation, if a patient is unstable, the decision to electrically cardiovert him/her should be made.

With wide complex tachyarrhythmias or ventricular tachyarrhythmias, in general most are highly unstable and cause the patient significant distress and would be electrically converted. However one notable exception is monomorphic ventricular tachycardia which patients may tolerate but can be treated pharmacologically with amiodarone or lidocaine.

Above all, the treatment modality is tailored to the individual, and varies based on the mechanism of the tachycardia (where it is originating from within the heart), on the duration of the tachycardia, how well the individual is tolerating the fast heart rate, the likelihood of recurrence once the rhythm is terminated, and any co-morbid conditions the individual is suffering from.

See also

- Vagus reflex
- Bradycardia, opposite of tachycardia

External links

- Dysautonomia Youth Network of America, Inc. [7]
- Postural Orthostatic Tachycardia Syndrome - overview from Dysautonomia Information Network [8]
- Heart Arrhythmias Respond to Ablation [9] UCLA Healthcare
- Heart Rate Calculator [10] Heart Rate Calculator for Diagnosis of Tachycardia

Pallor

ICD-10	R 23.1 [1]
ICD-9	782.61 [2]

Pallor is a reduced amount of oxyhemoglobin in skin or mucous membrane, a pale color which can be caused by illness, emotional shock or stress, stimulant use, lack of exposure to sunlight, anemia or genetics. It is more evident on the face and palms. It can develop suddenly or gradually, depending on the cause.

Pallor is not usually clinically significant unless it is accompanied by a general pallor (pale lips, tongue, palms, mouth and other regions with mucous membranes). It is distinguished from similar symptoms such as hypopigmentation (loss of skin pigment).

Pale skin is also a very light skin tone most commonly associated with people of European descent, particularly people of Celtic and Scandinavian descent. In addition, people who avoid sun exposure and thus avoid sun tanning also tend to have paler complexions in comparison to their peers.

Possible causes

- migraine attack or headache
- natural genetics
- excess estradiol and/or estrone
- vitamin D deficiency
- lack of sun tanning
- weight gain
- osteoporosis
- emotional response, due to fear, embarrassment, grief
- anemia, due to blood loss, poor nutrition, or underlying disease such as sickle cell anemia
- shock, a medical emergency caused by illness or injury
- frostbite
- cancer
- hypoglycemia
- leukemia
- albinism
- panic attack
- heart disease
- hypothyroidism

- hypopituitarism
- scurvy
- shock (medical)
- tuberculosis
- sleep deprivation
- depression
- pheochromocytoma
- squeamishness
- visceral larval migrans
- High doses or chronic use of amphetamines
- Reaction to ethanol and/or other drugs such as cannabis
- Lead poisoning

Depression (mood)

Depression is a state of low mood and aversion to activity. Depressed people may feel sad, anxious, empty, hopeless, helpless, worthless, guilty, irritable or restless. They may lose interest in activities that once were pleasurable, experience loss of appetite or overeating, or problems concentrating, remembering details or making decisions; and may contemplate or attempt suicide. Insomnia, excessive sleeping, fatigue, loss of energy, or aches, pains or digestive problems that are resistant to treatment may be present.

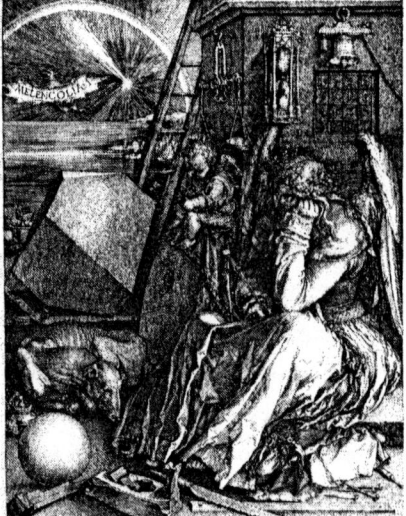

Albrecht Dürer's engraving *Melencolia I*, ca. 1514

Illnesses featuring depression

Psychiatric syndromes

A number of psychiatric syndromes feature depressed mood as a main symptom. Mood disorders are a group of disorders considered to be primary disturbances of mood. Within them, major depressive disorder (MDD), commonly called major depression, or clinical depression, is a condition where a person has at least two weeks of depressed mood or a loss of interest or pleasure in nearly all activities. Dysthymia is a state of chronic depressed mood, the symptoms of which do not meet the severity of a major depressive episode. People suffering bipolar disorder may also experience major depressive episodes.

Outside the mood disorders, dysthymia is also commonly a feature of borderline personality disorder. Adjustment disorder with depressed mood is a mood disturbance appearing as a psychological response to an identifiable event or stressor, in which the resulting emotional or behavioral symptoms are significant but do not meet the criteria for a major depressive episode.

Non-psychiatric illnesses

Depressed mood can be the result of a number of infectious diseases and physiological problems. For example, mononucleosis, which can be caused by two different viral infections, often results in symptoms that mimic a depressive psychiatric disorder; and depression is often one of the early symptoms of hypothyroidism. For a discussion of non-psychiatric medical illnesses that can cause depressed mood, see Depression (differential diagnoses).

Prevalence

On October 1, 2010 the U.S. Centers for Disease Control and Prevention (CDC) released a report regarding the prevalence of current depression in the United States during 2006 and 2008 based on an analysis of Behavioral Risk Factor Surveillance System (BRFSS) survey data from 2006 and 2008. Current depression was defined as meeting BRFSS criteria for either major depression or "other depression" during the 2 weeks preceding the survey. The report summarizes the results of that analysis, which indicated that, among 235,067 adults (in 45 states, the District of Columbia [DC], Puerto Rico, and the U.S. Virgin Islands), 9.0% met the criteria for current depression, including 3.4% who met the criteria for major depression. By state, age-standardized estimates for current depression ranged from 4.8% in North Dakota to 14.8% in Mississippi.

Physiology or mechanism

Depression is associated with changes in substances in the brain (neurotransmitters) that help nerve cells communicate, such as serotonin, dopamine and norepinephrine. The levels of these neurotransmitters can be influenced by, among other things, physical illnesses, genetics, hormonal changes, medications, aging, brain injuries, seasonal/light cycle changes, and social circumstances.

Assessment

A full patient medical history, physical assessment, and thorough evaluation of symptoms helps determine the cause of the depression. Standardized questionnaires can be helpful such as the Hamilton Rating Scale for Depression, and the Beck Depression Inventory.

A doctor generally performs a medical examination and selected investigations to rule out other causes of symptoms. These include blood tests measuring TSH and thyroxine to exclude hypothyroidism; basic electrolytes and serum calcium to rule out a metabolic disturbance; and a full blood count including ESR to rule out a systemic infection or chronic disease. Adverse affective reactions to medications or alcohol misuse are often ruled out, as well. Testosterone levels may be evaluated to diagnose hypogonadism, a cause of depression in men.

Subjective cognitive complaints appear in older depressed people, but they can also be indicative of the onset of a dementing disorder, such as Alzheimer's disease. Cognitive testing and brain imaging can help distinguish depression from dementia. A CT scan can exclude brain pathology in those with psychotic, rapid-onset or otherwise unusual symptoms. Investigations are not generally repeated for a subsequent episode unless there is a medical indication.

See also

- Rational depression

References

Selected cited works

- American Psychiatric Association. *Diagnostic and statistical manual of mental disorders, Fourth Edition, Text Revision: DSM-IV-TR*. Washington, DC: American Psychiatric Publishing, Inc.; 2000a. ISBN 0890420254.

Weakness

"Asthenia" redirects here. The tortrix moth genus is nowadays considered a junior synonym of Epinotia.

ICD-10	M 62.8 [1]
ICD-9	728.87 [2] (728.9 [3] before 10/01/03)
DiseasesDB	22832 [4]
MedlinePlus	003174 [5]
MeSH	D018908 [6]

Weakness is a symptom used to describe a number of different conditions, including: lack of muscle strength, malaise, dizziness or fatigue. The causes are many and can be divided into conditions that have true or perceived muscle weakness. True muscle weakness is a primary symptom of a variety of skeletal muscle diseases, including muscular dystrophy and inflammatory myopathy. It occurs in neuromuscular junction disorders, such as myasthenia gravis.

Definition

Weakness is used to describe a number of symptoms including: loss of muscle strength, malaise, dizziness or fatigue. The term can be divided into two other more specific states, *true weakness* and *perceived weakness*.

- **True weakness** (or **neuromuscular**) describes a condition where the force exerted by the muscles is less than would be expected, for example muscular dystrophy.
- **Perceived weakness** (or **non-neuromuscular**) describes a condition where a person feels more effort than normal is required to exert a given amount of force but actual muscle strength is normal, for example chronic fatigue syndrome.

In some conditions, such as myasthenia gravis muscle strength is normal when resting, but *true weakness* occurs after the muscle has been subjected to exercise. This is also true for some cases of CSI, where objective post-exertion muscle weakness with delayed recovery time has been measured and is a feature of some of the published definitions.

- **Asthenia** (Greek: ασθένεια, lit. *lack of strength* but also *disease*) is a medical term denoting symptoms of physical weakness and loss of strength.

A condition in which the body lacks or has lost strength either as a whole or in any of its parts. General asthenia occurs in many chronic wasting diseases, such as anemia and cancer, and is probably most marked in diseases of the adrenal gland. Asthenia may be limited to certain organs or systems of organs, as in asthenopia, characterized by ready fatiguability.

Asthenia is also a side effect of some medications and treatments, such as Ritonavir (a protease inhibitor used in HIV treatment), vaccines such as the HPV vaccine Gardasil and fentanyl patches (an opioid used to treat pain).

The condition is also commonly seen in patients suffering from chronic fatigue syndrome, sleep disorders or chronic disorders of the heart, lungs or kidneys.

Differentiating between psychogenic asthenia and true asthenia with muscular weakness is often difficult, and in time apparent psychogenic asthenia accompanying many chronic disorders is seen to progress into a primary weakness.

Differential diagnosis

Weakness can be central, neural and peripheral. Central muscle weakness manifests as an overall, bodily or systemic, sense of energy deprivation, and peripheral weakness manifests as a local, muscle-specific incapacity to do work. Neural weakness can be both central and peripheral.

Central

The central component to muscle fatigue is generally described in terms of a reduction in the neural drive or nerve-based motor command to working muscles that results in a decline in the force output. It has been suggested that the reduced neural drive during exercise may be a protective mechanism to prevent organ failure if the work was continued at the same intensity. The exact mechanisms of central fatigue are unknown although there has been a great deal of interest in the role of serotonergic pathways.

Neural

Nerves are responsible for controlling the contraction of muscles, determining the number, sequence and force of muscular contraction. Most movements require a force far below what a muscle could in potential generate, and barring pathology nervous fatigue is seldom an issue. For extremely powerful contractions that are close to the upper limit of a muscle's ability to generate force, nervous fatigue can be a limiting factor in untrained individuals. In novice strength trainers, the muscle's ability to generate force is most strongly limited by nerve's ability to sustain a high-frequency signal. After a period of maximum contraction, the nerve's signal reduces in frequency and the force generated by the contraction diminishes. There is no sensation of pain or discomfort, the muscle appears to simply 'stop listening' and gradually cease to move, often going backwards. As there is insufficient stress on the muscles and tendons, there will often be no delayed onset muscle soreness following the workout. Part of the process of strength training is increasing the nerve's ability to generate sustained, high frequency signals which allow a muscle to contract with their greatest force. It is this neural training that causes several weeks worth of rapid gains in strength, which level off once the nerve is generating maximum contractions and the muscle reaches its physiological limit. Past this point, training effects increase muscular strength through myofibrilar or sarcoplasmic hypertrophy and metabolic fatigue becomes the factor limiting contractile force.

Peripheral

Peripheral muscle fatigue during physical work is considered an inability for the body to supply sufficient energy or other metabolites to the contracting muscles to meet the increased energy demand. This is the most common case of physical fatigue—affecting a national average of 72% of adults in the work force in 2002. This causes contractile dysfunction that is manifested in the eventual reduction or lack of ability of a single muscle or local group of muscles to do work. The insufficiency of energy, i.e. sub-optimal aerobic metabolism, generally results in the accumulation of lactic acid and other acidic anaerobic metabolic by-products in the muscle, causing the stereotypical burning sensation of local muscle fatigue, though recent studies have indicated otherwise, actually finding that lactic acid is a source of energy.

The fundamental difference between the peripheral and central theories of muscle fatigue is that the peripheral model of muscle fatigue assumes failure at one or more sites in the chain that initiates muscle contraction. Peripheral regulation is therefore dependent on the localised metabolic chemical conditions of the local muscle affected, whereas the central model of muscle fatigue is an integrated mechanism that works to preserve the integrity of the system by initiating muscle fatigue through muscle derecruitment, based on collective feedback from the periphery, before cellular or organ failure occurs. Therefore the feedback that is read by this central regulator could include chemical and mechanical as well as cognitive cues. The significance of each of these factors will depend on the nature of the fatigue-inducing work that is being performed.

Though not universally used, 'metabolic fatigue' is a common alternative term for peripheral muscle weakness, because of the reduction in contractile force due to the direct or indirect effects of the reduction of substrates or accumulation of metabolites within the muscle fiber. This can occur through a simple lack of energy to fuel contraction, or interference with the ability of Ca^{2+} to stimulate actin and myosin to contract.

Lactic acid

It was once believed that lactic acid build-up was the cause of muscle fatigue. The assumption was lactic acid had a "pickling" effect on muscles, inhibiting their ability to contract. The impact of lactic acid on performance is now uncertain, it may assist or hinder muscle fatigue.

Produced as a by-product of fermentation, lactic acid can increase intracellular acidity of muscles. This can lower the sensitivity of contractile apparatus to Ca^{2+} but also has the effect of increasing cytoplasmic Ca^{2+} concentration through an inhibition of the chemical pump that actively transports calcium out of the cell. This counters inhibiting effects of K^+ on muscular action potentials. Lactic acid also has a negating effect on the chloride ions in the muscles, reducing their inhibition of contraction and leaving potassium ions as the only restricting influence on muscle contractions, though the effects of potassium are much less than if there were no lactic acid to remove the chloride ions. Ultimately, it is uncertain if lactic acid reduces fatigue through increased intracellular calcium or increases fatigue through reduced sensitivity of contractile proteins to Ca^{2+}.

Associated conditions

Many different conditions can cause weakness. In 2010 DiagnosisPro listed 464 possible cause. True weakness may be due to problems with the nerves, neuromuscular junction or with muscles.

- Amyotrophic lateral sclerosis
- Botulism
- Centronuclear myopathy
- Myotubular myopathy
- Muscle Atrophy
- Sarcopenia
- Dysautonomia
- Charcot-Marie-Tooth
- Hypokalemia
- Motor neurone disease
- Muscular dystrophy
- Myotonic dystrophy
- Myasthenia gravis
- Progressive muscular atrophy
- Spinal muscular atrophy
- Cerebral palsy
- Infectious mononucleosis
- Herpes zoster
- Vitamin D deficiency
- Fibromyalgia

- Celiac disease
- Hypercortisolism (Cushing's syndrome)
- Hypocortisolism (Addison's disease)
- Primary hyperaldosteronism (Conn's syndrome)
- Ehlers-Danlos syndrome
- Diarrhea
- McArdle's Disease
- Ross River Fever
- Barmah Forest Fever

Pathophysiology

Main article: muscle contraction

Muscle cells work by detecting a flow of electrical impulses from the brain which signals them to contract through the release of calcium by the sarcoplasmic reticulum. Fatigue (reduced ability to generate force) may occur due to the nerve, or within the muscle cells themselves. New research from scientists at Columbia University suggests that muscle fatigue is caused by calcium leaking out of the muscle cell. This causes there to be less calcium available for the muscle cell. In addition an enzyme is proposed to be activated by this released calcium which eats away at muscle fibers.

Substrates within the muscle generally serve to power muscular contractions. They include molecules such as adenosine triphosphate (ATP), glycogen and creatine phosphate. ATP binds to the myosin head and causes the 'ratchetting' that results in contraction according to the sliding filament model. Creatine phosphate stores energy so ATP can be rapidly regenerated within the muscle cells from adenosine diphosphate (ADP) and inorganic phosphate ions, allowing for sustained powerful contractions that last between 5–7 seconds. Glycogen is the intramuscular storage form of glucose, used to generate energy quickly once intramuscular creatine stores are exhausted, producing lactic acid as a metabolic byproduct. Contrary to common belief, lactic acid accumulation doesn't actually cause the burning sensation we feel when we exhaust our oxygen and oxidative metabolism, but in actuality, lactic acid in presence of oxygen recycles to produce pyruvate in the liver which is known as the Cori cycle.

Substrates produce metabolic fatigue by being depleted during exercise, resulting in a lack of intracellular energy sources to fuel contractions. In essence, the muscle stops contracting because it lacks the energy to do so.

External links

- Jun Mapili's Muscle Weakness Coding Checklist [7]
- AllRefer [8]
- Unexplained Muscle Weakness - Information About McArdle's Disease [9]

Dyspnea

ICD-10	R 06.0 [1]
ICD-9	786.0 [2]
DiseasesDB	15892 [3]
MedlinePlus	003075 [4]
MeSH	D004417 [5]

Dyspnea (also spelled **dyspnoea**) or (**shortness of breath** (SOB), **air hunger**), is the subjective symptom of *breathlessness*. It is a normal symptom of heavy exertion however becomes pathological if it occurs in unexpected situations. In 85% of cases it is due to either: asthma, pneumonia, cardiac ischemia, interstitial lung disease, congestive heart failure, chronic obstructive pulmonary disease, or psychogenic causes. Treatment typically depends on the underlying cause.

Definition

Lungs and breathing activity
Eupnea - normal breathing
Bradypnea - decreased breathing rate
Dyspnea or *shortness of breath* - sensation of respiratory distress
Hyperaeration/Hyperinflation - increased lung volume
Hyperpnea - faster and/or deeper breathing
Hyperventilation - increased breathing that causes CO_2 loss
Labored breathing - physical presentation of respiratory distress
Tachypnea - increased breathing rate

Dyspnea does not have a well defined or universally accepted definition. It is defined by the American Thoracic Society as the "subjective experience of breathing discomfort that consists of qualitatively distinct sensations that vary in intensity. The experience derives from interactions among multiple physiological, psychological, social, and environmental factors, and may induce secondary physiological and behavioral responses." Other definitions of dyspnea include: "difficulty in breathing" and "uncomfortable awareness of breathing", or simple "breathlessness".

Acute breathlessness is defined as severe shortness of breath that develops over minutes to hours. Chronic breathlessness on the other hand comes on over weeks or months.

Differential diagnosis

Main article: Differential diagnosis of dyspnea

While shortness of breath is generally caused by disorders of the cardiac or respiratory system other system such as musculoskeletal, endocrine, hematologic, and psychiatric maybe the cause. DiagnosisPro, an online medical expert system, listed 497 distinct causes in October of 2010. The most common cardiovascular causes are acute myocardial infarction and congestive heart failure while common pulmonary causes include: chronic obstructive pulmonary disease, asthma, pneumothorax, and pneumonia.

Acute coronary syndrome

Acute coronary syndrome frequently presents with retrosternal chest discomfort and difficulty catching the breath. It however may atypically present with shortness of breath alone. Risk factors include: old age, smoking, hypertension, hyperlipidemia, and diabetes. An electrocardiogram and cardiac enzymes are important both for diagnosis and directing treatment. Treatment involves measures to decrease the oxygen requirement of the heart and efforts to increase blood flow.

Congestive heart failure

Congestive heart failure frequently presents with SOB with exertion, orthopnea, and paroxysmal nocturnal dyspnea. It affects between 1-2% of the general United States population and occurs in 10% of those over 65 years old. Risk factors for acute decompensation include: high dietary salt intake, medication noncompliance, cardiac ischemia, dysrhythmias, renal failure, pulmonary emboli, hypertension, and infections. Treatment efforts are directed towards decreasing lung congestion.

Chronic obstructive pulmonary disease

People with chronic obstructive pulmonary disease (COPD), most commonly emphysema or chronic bronchitis, frequently have chronic shortness of breath and a chronic productive cough. An acute exacerbation presents with increased shortness of breath and sputum production. COPD is a risk factor for pneumothorax thus this condition should be ruled out. In an acute exacerbation treatment is with a combination of anticholinergics, beta$_2$-adrenoceptor agonists, steroids and possibly positive pressure ventilation.

Asthma

Asthma is the most common reason for presenting to the emergency with shortness of breath. It is the most common long disease in both developing and developed countries affecting about 5% of the population. Other symptoms include: wheezing, tightness in the chest, and a non productive cough. Inhaled beta2-adrenergic agonist (salbutamol) are first line therapy and usually lead to prompt improvement.

Pneumothorax

Pneumothorax presents typically with pleuritic chest pain of acute onset and shortness of breath not improved with oxygen. Physical findings may include: absent breath sounds on one side of the chest, jugular venous distension, and tracheal deviation.

Pneumonia

The symptoms of pneumonia are fever, productive cough, shortness of breath, and pleuritic chest pain. Inspiratory crackles may be heard on exam. A chest x-ray can be useful to differential pneumonia from congestive heart failure. As the cause is usually a bacterial infections antibiotics are typically used for treatment.

Pulmonary embolism

Pulmonary embolism classically presents with an acute onset of shortness of breath. Other presenting symptoms include: pleuritic chest pain,cough, hemoptysis, and fever. Risk factors include: deep vein thrombosis, recent surgery, cancer, and previous thromboembolism. It must always be considered in those with acute onset of shortness of breath due to its high risk of mortality. Diagnosis however may be difficult. Treatment is typically with anticoagulants.

Other

Other important or common causes of shortness of breath include: cardiac tamponade, anemia, anaphylaxis, interstitial lung disease and panic attacks. Cardiac tamponade presents with dyspnea, tachycardia, elevated jugular venous pressure, and pulsus paradoxus. The gold standard for diagnosis is ultrasound. Anemia, that develops gradually, usually presents with exertional dyspnea, fatigue, weakness, and tachycardia. It may lead to heart failure. Anaphylaxis typically begins over a few minutes in a person with a previous history of the same. Other symptoms include: urticaria, throat swelling, and gastrointestinal upset. The primary treatment is epinephrine. Interstitial lung disease presents with gradual onset of shortness of breath typically with a history of a predisposing environmental exposure. Shortness of breath is often the only symptom in those with tachydysrhythmias. Panic attacks typically present with hyperventilation, sweating, and numbness. They are however a diagnosis of exclusion.

Pathophysiology

A number of different physiological pathway may lead to shortness of breath including via chemoreceptors, mechanoreceptors, and lung receptors.

It is currently thought that there are three main components that contribute to dyspnea: afferent signals, efferent signals, and central information processing. It is believed that the central processing in the brain compares the afferent and efferent signals, and that a "mismatch" results in the sensation of dyspnea. In other words, dyspnea may result when the need for ventilation (afferent signaling) is not being met by the physical breathing that is occurring (efferent signaling). Afferent signals are sensory neuronal signals that ascend to the brain. Afferent neurons significant in dyspnea arise from a large number of sources including the carotid bodies, medulla, lungs, and chest wall. Chemoreceptors in the carotid bodies and medulla supply information regarding the blood gas levels of O_2, CO_2 and H^+. In the lungs, juxtacapillary (J) receptors are sensitive to pulmonary interstitial edema, while stretch receptors signal bronchoconstriction. Muscle spindles in the chest wall signal the stretch and tension of the respiratory muscles. Thus, poor ventilation leading to hypercapnia, left heart failure leading to interstitial edema (impairing gas exchange), asthma causing bronchoconstriction (limiting airflow) and muscle fatigue leading to ineffective respiratory muscle action could all contribute to a feeling of dyspnea.

Efferent signals are the motor neuronal signals descending to the respiratory muscles. The most important respiratory muscle is the diaphragm. Other respiratory muscles include the external and internal intercostal muscles, the abdominal muscles and the accessory breathing muscles.

As the brain receives its plentiful supply of afferent information relating to ventilation, it is able to compare it to the current level of respiration as determined by the efferent signals. If the level of respiration is inappropriate for the body's status then dyspnea might occur. It is worth noting that there is a psychological component of dyspnea as well, as some people may become aware of their breathing in such circumstances but not experience the distress typical of dyspnea.

Evaluation

MRC Breathlessness Scale

Grade	Degree of dyspnea
0	no dyspnea except with strenuous exercise
1	dyspnea when walking up an incline or hurrying on the level
2	walks slower than most on the level, or stops after 15 minutes of walking on the level
3	stops after a few minutes of walking on the level
4	with minimal activity such as getting dressed, too dyspneic to leave the house

The initial approach to evaluation begins by assessment of the airway, breathing, and circulation followed by a medical history and physical examination. Signs that represent significant severity include: hypotension, hypoxemia, tracheal deviation, altered mental status, unstable dysrhythmia, stridor, intercostal indrawing, cyanosis, and absent breath sounds.

A number of scales may be used to quantify the degree of shortness of breath. It may be subjectively rated on a scale from 1 to 10 with descriptors associated with the number (The Modified Borg Scale). Alternatively a scale such as the MRC Breathlessness Scale might be used - it suggests five different grades of dyspnea based on the circumstances in which it arises.

Blood tests

A number of labs maybe helpful in determining the cause of shortness of breath. D-dimer while useful to rule out a pulmonary embolism in those who are at low risk is not of much value if it is positive as it may be positive in a number of conditions that lead to shortness of breath. A low level of brain natriuretic peptide is useful in ruling out congestive heart failure however a high level while supportive of the diagnosis could also be due to advanced age, renal failure, acute coronary syndrome, or a large pulmonary embolism.

Imaging

A chest x-ray is useful to confirm or rule out a pneumothorax, pulmonary edema, or pneumonia. Spiral computed tomography with intravenousradiocontrast is the imaging study of choice to evaluate for pulmonary embolism.

Treatment

In those who are none palliative the primary treatment of shortness of breath is directed at its underlying cause. Extra oxygen is effective in those with hypoxia however has no effect in those with normal blood oxygen saturations.

Palliative

Along with the measure above systemic immediate release opioids are beneficial in reducing the symptom of shortness of breath due to both cancer and non cancer causes. There is a lack of evidence to recommend midazolam, nebulised opioids, the use of gas mixtures, or cognitive-behavioral therapy.

Epidemiology

People with SOB make up about 7% of people who present to the emergency department in the United States. Of these approximately 51% are admitted to hospital and 13% are dead within a year. Some studies have suggested that up to 27% of people suffer from dyspnea, while in dying patients 75% will experience it. Acute shortness of breath is the most common reason people who are palliative visit an emergency department.

Etymology

Dyspnea (pronounced /dɪspˈniːə/ *disp-NEE-ə*), (from Latin *dyspnoea*, from Greek *dyspnoia* from *dyspnoos*) literally means disordered breathing.

External links

- *Dyspnea* [6] at GPnotebook

Neuropathic pain

Neuropathic pain is pain arising as a direct consequence of a lesion or disease affecting the somatosensory system. Neuropathic pain cannot be explained by a single disease process or a single specific location of damage.

It may be associated with abnormal sensations called dysesthesias, which occur spontaneously and allodynia that occurs in response to external stimuli. Neuropathic pain may have continuous and/or episodic (paroxysmal) components. The latter are likened to an electric shock. Common qualities include burning or coldness, "pins and needles" sensations, numbness and itching. Nociceptive pain is more commonly described as aching.

Up to 7% to 8% of the population is affected and in 5% of persons it may be severe. Neuropathic pain may result from disorders of the peripheral nervous system or the central nervous system (brain and spinal cord). Thus, neuropathic pain may be divided into peripheral neuropathic pain, central neuropathic pain, or mixed (peripheral and central) neuropathic pain.

Central neuropathic pain is found in spinal cord injury, multiple sclerosis, and some strokes. Fibromyalgia, a disorder of chronic widespread pain, is potentially a central pain disorder and is responsive to medications that are effective for neuropathic pain.

Aside from diabetes (see Diabetic neuropathy) and other metabolic conditions, the common causes of painful peripheral neuropathies are herpes zoster infection, HIV-related neuropathies, nutritional deficiencies, toxins, remote manifestations of malignancies, genetic, and immune mediated disorders or physical trauma to a nerve trunk.

Neuropathic pain is common in cancer as a direct result of cancer on peripheral nerves (e.g., compression by a tumor), or as a side effect of chemotherapy , radiation injury or surgery.

Mechanisms

The starting point for neuropathic pain is a lesion or dysfunction within the somatosensory system. Current knowledge regarding the mechanisms of neuropathic pain is incomplete and is biased by a focus on animal models of peripheral nerve injury.

Peripheral

Under normal circumstances, pain sensations are carried by unmyelinated and thinly myelinated nerve fibers, designated C-fibers and A-delta fibers, respectively. After a peripheral nerve lesion, aberrant regeneration may occur. Neurons become unusually sensitive and develop spontaneous pathological activity, abnormal excitability, and heightened sensitivity to chemical, thermal and mechanical stimuli. This phenomenon is called "peripheral sensitization".

Central

The dorsal horn neurons give rise to the spinothalamic tract (STT), which constitutes the major ascending nociceptive pathway. As a consequence of ongoing spontaneous activity arising in the periphery, STT neurons develop an increased background activity, enlarged receptive field and increased responses to afferent impulses, including normally innocuous tactile stimuli. This phenomenon is called central sensitization. Central sensitization has been proposed as an important mechanism of persistent neuropathic pain.

Other mechanisms, however, may take place at the central level after peripheral nerve damage. The loss of afferent signals induces functional changes in dorsal horn neurons. A decrease in the large fiber input decreases activity of interneurons inhibiting nociceptive neurons i.e. loss of afferent inhibition. Hypoactivity of the descending antinociceptive systems or loss of descending inhibition may be another factor. With loss of neuronal input (deafferentation) the STT neurons begin to fire spontaneously, a phenomenon designated "deafferentation hypersensitivity."

Non-neural glial cells may play a role in central sensitization. Peripheral nerve injury induces glial to releasing glial proinflammatory cytokines and glutamate which, in turn influence neurons.

Mechanisms at light-microscopic and submicroscopic levels

The phenomenon described above are dependent on changes at light-microscopic and submicroscopic levels. Altered expression of ion channels, changes in neurotransmitters and their receptors as well as altered gene expression in response to neural input are at play.

Treatments

Neuropathic pain can be very difficult to treat with only some 40-60% of patients achieving partial relief.

In addition to the work of Dworkin, O'Connor and Backonja et al., cited above, there have been several recent attempts to derive guidelines for pharmacological therapy. These have combined evidence from randomized controlled trials with expert opinion.

Determining the best treatment for individual patients remains challenging. Attempts to translate scientific studies into best practices are limited by factors such as differences in reference populations and a lack of head-to-head studies. Furthermore, multi-drug combinations and the needs of special populations, such as children, require more study.

It is common practice in medicine to designate classes of medication according to their most common or familiar use e.g. as "antidepressants" and "anti-epileptic drugs" (AED's). These drugs have alternate uses to treat pain because the human nervous system employs common mechanisms for different functions, for example ion channels for impulse generation and neurotransmitters for cell-to-cell signaling.

Favored treatments are certain antidepressants e.g. tricyclics and selective serotonin-norepinephrine re-uptake inhibitors (SNRI's), anticonvulsants, especially pregabalin (Lyrica) and gabapentin (Neurontin), and topical lidocaine. Opioid analgesics and tramadol are recognized as useful agents but are not recommended as first line treatments. Many of the pharmacologic treatments for chronic neuropathic pain decrease the sensitivity of nociceptive receptors, or desensitize C fibers such that they transmit fewer signals.

Some drugs may exert their influence through descending pain modulating pathways. These descending pain modulating pathways originate in the brainstem.

Antidepressants

Main article: Antidepressants

The functioning of antidepressants is different in neuropathic pain from that observed in depression. Activation of descending norepinephrinergic and serotonergic pathways to the spinal cord limit pain signals ascending to the brain. Antidepressants will relieve neuropathic pain in non-depressed persons.

In animal models of neuropathic pain it has been found that compounds which only block serotonin reuptake do not improve neuropathic pain. Similarly, compounds that only block norepinephrine reuptake also do not improve neuropathic pain. Compounds such as duloxetine, venlafaxine, and milnacipran that block both serotonin reuptake and norepinephrine reuptake do improve neuropathic pain.

Bupropion has been found to have efficacy in the treatment of neuropathic pain.

Tricyclic antidepressants may also have effects on sodium channels.

Anticonvulsants

Main article: Anticonvulsants

Pregabalin (Lyrica) and gabapentin (Neurontin) work by blocking specific calcium channels on neurons. The actions of the anticonvulsants carbamazepine (Tegretol) and oxcarbazepine (Trileptal), especially effective on trigeminal neuralgia, are principally on sodium channels.

Lamotrigine may have a special role in treating two conditions for which there are few alternatives, namely post stroke pain and HIV/AIDS-related neuropathy in that subgroup on antiretroviral therapy.

Opioids

Main article: Opioids

Opioids, also known as narcotics, are increasingly recognized as important treatment options for chronic pain. They are not considered first line treatments in neuropathic pain but remain the most consistently effective class of drugs for this condition. Opioids must be used only in appropriate individuals and under close medical supervision.

Several opioids, particularly methadone, have NMDA antagonist activity in addition to their μ-opioid agonist properties.

Methadone and ketobemidone possess NMDA antagonism. Methadone does so because it is a racemic mixture; only the l-isomer is a potent μ-opioid agonist.

There is little evidence to indicate that one strong opioid is more effective than another. Expert opinion leans toward the use of methadone for neuropathic pain, in part because of NMDA antagonism. It is reasonable to base the choice of opioid on other factors.

Topical agents

In some forms of neuropathy, especially post-herpetic neuralgia, the topical application of local anesthetics such as lidocaine can provide relief. A transdermal patch containing lidocaine is available commercially in some countries.

Repeated topical applications of capsaicin, are followed by a prolonged period of reduced skin sensibility referred to as desensitization, or nociceptor inactivation. Capsaicin not only depletes substance P but also results in a reversible degeneration of epidermal nerve fibers. Nevertheless, benefits appear to be modest with standard (low) strength preparations.

Cannabinoids

Marijuana's active ingredients are called cannabinoids. Unfortunately, strongly held beliefs make discussion of the appropriate use of these substances, in a medical context, difficult. Similar considerations apply to opioids.

A recent study showed smoked marijuana is beneficial in treating symptoms of HIV-associated peripheral neuropathy. Nabilone is an artificial cannabinoid which is significantly more potent than delta-9-tetrahydrocannabinol (THC). Nabilone produces less relief of chronic neuropathic pain and had slightly more side effects than dihydrocodeine.

The predominant adverse effects are CNS depression and cardiovascular effects which are mild and well tolerated but, psychoactive side effects limit their use. A complicating issue may be a narrow therapeutic window; lower doses decrease pain but higher doses have the opposite effect.

Sativex, a fixed dose combination of delta-9-tetrahydrocannabinol (THC) and cannabidiol, is sold as an oromucosal spray. The product is approved in Canada as adjunctive treatment for the symptomatic relief of neuropathic pain in multiple sclerosis, and for cancer related pain.

Long-term studies are needed to assess the probability of weight gain, unwanted psychological influences and other adverse effects.

Botulinum Toxin Type A (Botox, BTX-A)

Main article: Botulinum toxin

Botulinum Toxin Type A (BTX-A) is best know by its trade name, Botox. Local intradermal injection of BTX-A is helpful in chronic focal painful neuropathies. The analgesic effects are not dependent on changes in muscle tone. Benefits persist for at least 14 weeks from the time of administration.

The utility of BTX-A in other painful conditions remains to be established.

NMDA antagonism

The *N*-methyl-D-aspartate (NMDA) receptor seems to play a major role in neuropathic pain and in the development of opioid tolerance. Dextromethorphan is an NMDA antagonist at high doses. Experiments in both animals and humans have established that NMDA antagonists such as ketamine and dextromethorphan can alleviate neuropathic pain and reverse opioid tolerance. Unfortunately, only a few NMDA antagonists are clinically available and their use is limited by unacceptable side effects.

Reducing sympathetic nervous stimulation

In some neuropathic pain syndromes, "crosstalk" occurs between descending sympathetic nerves and ascending sensory nerves. Increases in sympathetic nervous system activity result in an increase of pain; this is known as sympathetically-mediated pain.

Lesioning operations on the sympathetic branch of the autonomic nervous system are sometimes carried out.

Dietary supplements

There are two dietary supplements that have clinical evidence showing them to be effective treatments of diabetic neuropathy; alpha lipoic acid and benfotiamine.

A 2007 review of studies found that injected (parenteral) administration of alpha lipoic acid (ALA) was found to reduce the various symptoms of peripheral diabetic neuropathy. While some studies on orally administered ALA had suggested a reduction in both the positive symptoms of diabetic neuropathy (including stabbing and burning pain) as well as neuropathic deficits (paresthesia), the metanalysis showed "more conflicting data whether it improves sensory symptoms or just neuropathic deficits alone". There is some limited evidence that ALA is also helpful in some other non-diabetic neuropathies.

Benfotiamine is a lipid-soluble form of thiamine that has several placebo-controlled double-blind trials proving efficacy in treating neuropathy and various other diabetic comorbidities.

Other modalities

In addition to pharmacological treatment several other modalities are commonly recommended. While lacking adequate double blind trials, these have shown to reduce pain and improve patient quality of life for chronic neuropathic pain: chiropractic, yoga, massage, meditation, cognitive therapy, and prescribed exercise. Some pain management specialists will try acupuncture, with variable results.

Transcutaneous electrical nerve stimulation (TENS) may be worth considering in chronic neurogenic pain. TENS, with certain electrical waveforms, appears to have an acupuncture-like function.

Infrared photo therapy has been used to treat neuropathic symptoms. However, recent work has cast doubt on the value of this approach.

Neuromodulators

Neuromodulation is a field of science, medicine and bioengineering that encompasses both implantable and non-implantable technologies (electrical and chemical) for treatment purposes.

Implanted devices are expensive and carry the risk of complications. Available studies have focused on conditions having a different prevalence than neuropathic pain patients in general. More research is needed to define the range of conditions for which they might be beneficial.

Spinal cord stimulators and implanted spinal pumps

Spinal cord stimulators, use electrodes placed adjacent to, but outside the spinal cord. The overall complication rate is one-third, most commonly due to lead migration or breakage. Lack of pain relief sometimes prompts device removal.

Infusion pumps deliver medication directly to the fluid filled (subarachnoid) space surrounding the spinal cord. Opioids alone or opioids with adjunctive medication (either a local anesthetic or clonidine) or more recently ziconotide are infused. Complications such as, serious infection (meningitis), urinary retention, hormonal disturbance and intrathecal granuloma formation have been noted.

There are no randomized studies of infusion pumps. For selected patients 50% or greater pain relief is achieved in 38% to 56% at six months but declines with the passage of time. These results must be viewed skeptically since placebo effects cannot be evaluated.

Motor cortex stimulation

Stimulation of the primary motor cortex through electrodes placed within the skull but outside the thick meningeal membrane (dura) has been used to treat pain. The level of stimulation is below that for motor stimulation. As compared with spinal stimulation, which requires a noticeable tingling (paresthesia) for benefit, the only palpable effect is pain relief.

Deep brain stimulation

The best long-term results with deep brain stimulation have been reported with targets in the periventricular/periaqueductal grey matter (79%), or the periventricular/periaqueductal grey matter plus thalamus and/or internal capsule (87%). There is a significant complication rate which increase over time.

Diarrhea

See also: Gastroenteritis

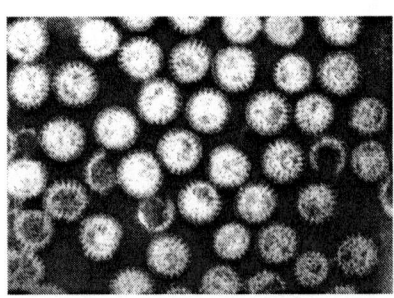

An electron micrograph of rotavirus, the cause of nearly 40% of hospitalizations from diarrhea in children under 5.

ICD-10	A 09. [1], K 59.1 [2]
ICD-9	787.91 [3]
DiseasesDB	3742 [4]
eMedicine	ped/583 [5]
MeSH	D003967 [6]

Diarrhea (from the Greek, διάρροια meaning "flowing through"), also spelled **diarrhoea**, is the condition of having three or more loose or liquid bowel movements per day. It is a common cause of death in developing countries and the second most common cause of infant deaths worldwide. The loss of fluids through diarrhea can cause dehydration and electrolyte imbalances. In 2009 diarrhea was estimated to have caused 1.1 million deaths in people aged 5 and over and 1.5 million deaths in children under the age of 5. Oral rehydration salts and zinc tablets are the treatment of choice and have been estimated to have saved 50 million children in the past 25 years.

Definition

Diarrhea is defined by the World Health Organization as having 3 or more loose or liquid stools per day, or as having more stools than is normal for that person.

Secretory

Secretory diarrhea means that there is an increase in the active secretion, or there is an inhibition of absorption. There is little to no structural damage. The most common cause of this type of diarrhea is a cholera toxin that stimulates the secretion of anions, especially chloride ions. Therefore, to maintain a charge balance in the lumen, sodium is carried with it, along with water. In this type of diarrhea intestinal fluid secretion is isotonic with plasma even during fasting. It continues even when there is no oral food intake.

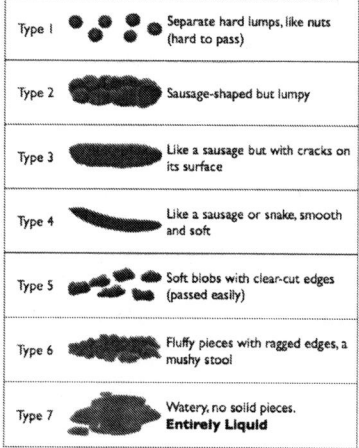

Type 7 on the Bristol Stool Chart indicate diarrhea

Osmotic

Osmotic diarrhea occurs when too much water is drawn into the bowels. This can be the result of maldigestion (e.g., pancreatic disease or celiac disease), in which the nutrients are left in the lumen to pull in water. Osmotic diarrhea can also be caused by osmotic laxatives (which work to alleviate constipation by drawing water into the bowels). In healthy individuals, too much magnesium or vitamin C or undigested lactose can produce osmotic diarrhea and distention of the bowel. A person who has lactose intolerance can have difficulty absorbing lactose after an extraordinarily high intake of dairy products. In persons who have fructose malabsorption, excess fructose intake can also cause diarrhea. High-fructose foods that also have a high glucose content are more absorbable and less likely to cause diarrhea. Sugar alcohols such as sorbitol (often found in sugar-free foods) are difficult for the body to absorb and, in large amounts, may lead to osmotic diarrhea. Diarrhea stops when offending agent (e.g. milk, sorbitol) is stopped.

Exudative

Exudative diarrhea occurs with the presence of blood and pus in the stool. This occurs with inflammatory bowel diseases, such as Crohn's disease or ulcerative colitis, and other severe infections such as *E. coli* or other forms of food poisoning.

Motility-related

Motility-related diarrhea is caused by the rapid movement of food through the intestines (hypermotility). If the food moves too quickly through the gastrointestinal tract, there is not enough time for sufficient nutrients and water to be absorbed. This can be due to a vagotomy or diabetic neuropathy, or a complication of menstruation[citation needed]. Hyperthyroidism can produce hypermotility and lead to pseudodiarrhea and occasionally real diarrhea. Diarrhea can be treated with antimotility agents (such as loperamide). Hypermotility can be observed in people who have had portions of their bowel removed, allowing less total time for absorption of nutrients.

Inflammatory

Inflammatory diarrhea occurs when there is damage to the mucosal lining or brush border, which leads to a passive loss of protein-rich fluids, and a decreased ability to absorb these lost fluids. Features of all three of the other types of diarrhea can be found in this type of diarrhea. It can be caused by bacterial infections, viral infections, parasitic infections, or autoimmune problems such as inflammatory bowel diseases. It can also be caused by tuberculosis, colon cancer, and enteritis. [citation needed]

Dysentery

Generally, if there is blood visible in the stools, it is not diarrhea, but dysentery. The blood an invasion of bowel tissue. Dysentery is a symptom of, among others, *Shigella*, *Entamoeba histolytica*, and *Salmonella*.

Differential diagnosis

Diarrhea is most commonly due to viral gastroenteritis with rotavirus accounting for 40% of cases in children under five.(p. 17) In travelers however bacterial infections predominate.

It can also be the part of the presentations of a number of medical conditions such as: Crohn's disease or mushroom poisoning.

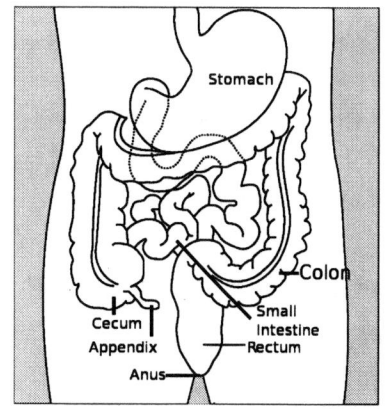

Diagram of the human gastrointestinal tract.

Infections

Main article: Infectious diarrhea

There are many causes of infectious diarrhea, which include viruses, bacteria and parasites. Norovirus is the most common cause of viral diarrhea in adults, but rotavirus is the most common cause in children under five years old. Adenovirus types 40 and 41, and astroviruses cause a significant number of infections.

The bacterium campylobacter is a common cause of bacterial diarrhea, but infections by salmonellae, shigellae and some strains of *Escherichia coli* (E.coli) are frequent. In the elderly, particularly those who have been treated with antibiotics for unrelated infections, a toxin produced by *Clostridium difficile* often causes severe diarrhea.

Parasites do not often cause diarrhea except for the protozoan *Giardia*, which can cause chronic infections if these are not diagnosed and treated with drugs such as metronidazole, and *Entamoeba histolytica*.

Other infectious agents such as parasites and bacterial toxins also occur. In sanitary living conditions where there is ample food and a supply of clean water, an otherwise healthy person usually recovers from viral infections in a few days. However, for ill or malnourished individuals, diarrhea can lead to severe dehydration and can become life-threatening.

Malabsorption

Main article: Malabsorption

Malabsorption is the inability to absorb food, mostly in the small bowel but also due to the pancreas.

Causes include:

- enzyme deficiencies or mucosal abnormality, as in food allergy and food intolerance, (e.g. celiac disease (gluten intolerance), lactose intolerance (intolerance to milk sugar, common in non-Europeans), fructose malabsorption)
- pernicious anemia (impaired bowel function due to the inability to absorb vitamin B_{12}),
- loss of pancreatic secretions (may be due to cystic fibrosis or pancreatitis),
- structural defects, like short bowel syndrome (surgically removed bowel) and radiation fibrosis (usually following cancer treatment and other drugs, including agents used in chemotherapy),
- certain drugs (like orlistat, which inhibits the absorption of fat).

Inflammatory bowel disease

Main article: Inflammatory bowel disease

The two overlapping types here are of unknown origin:

- Ulcerative colitis is marked by chronic bloody diarrhea and inflammation mostly affects the distal colon near the rectum.
- Crohn's disease typically affects fairly well demarcated segments of bowel in the colon and often affects the end of the small bowel.

Irritable bowel syndrome

Main article: Irritable bowel syndrome

Another possible cause of diarrhea is irritable bowel syndrome (IBS) which usually presents with abdominal discomfort relieved by defecation and unusual stool (diarrhea or constipation) for at least 3 days a week over the previous 3 months. There is no direct treatment for IBS, however symptoms can be managed through a combination of dietary changes, soluble fiber supplements, and/or medications.

Other causes

- Diarrhea can be caused by chronic ethanol ingestion.
- Ischemic bowel disease. This usually affects older people and can be due to blocked arteries.
- Hormone-secreting tumors: some hormones (e.g., serotonin) can cause diarrhea if excreted in excess (usually from a tumor).
- Chronic mild diarrhea in infants and toddlers may occur with no obvious cause and with no other ill effects; this condition is called toddler's diarrhea.

Pathophysiology

Evolution

According to two researchers, Nesse and Williams, diarrhea may function as an evolved expulsion defense mechanism. As a result, if it is stopped, there might be a delay in recovery. They cite in support of this argument research published in 1973 which found that treating *Shigella* with the anti-diarrhea drug (Co-phenotrope, Lomotil) caused people to stay feverish twice as long as those not so treated. The researchers indeed themselves observed that: "Lomotil may be contraindicated in shigellosis. Diarrhea may represent a defense mechanism".

Diagnostic approach

The following types of diarrhea may indicate further investigation is needed:

- In infants
- Moderate or severe diarrhea in young children
- Associated with blood
- Continues for more than two days
- Associated non cramping abdominal pain, fever, weight loss, etc.
- In travelers
- In food handlers, because of the potential to infect others;
- In institutions such as hospitals, child care centers, or geriatric and convalescent homes.

A severity score is used to aid diagnosis in children.

Prevention

A rotavirus vaccine has the potential to decrease rates of diarrhea. There are currently two licensed vaccines against rotavirus. New vaccines against rotavirus, *Shigella*, ETEC, and cholera are under development, as well as other causes of infectious diarrhea.

Management

In many cases of diarrhea, replacing lost fluid and salts is the only treatment needed. This is usually by mouth – oral rehydration therapy – or, in severe cases, intravenously. Diet restrictions such as the BRAT diet are no longer recommended. Research does not support the limiting of milk to children as doing so has no effect on duration of diarrhea.

Medications such as loperamide (Imodium), bismuth subsalicylate may be beneficial, however they may be contraindicated in certain situations.

Medications

Antibiotics

While antibiotics are beneficial in certain type of acute diarrhea they are usually not used except in specific situations. There are concerns that antibiotic may increase the risk of hemolytic uremic syndrome in people infected with Escherichia coli O157:H7. In resource poor countries treatment with antibiotics may be beneficial. However, some bacteria are developing antibiotic resistance, particularly *Shigella*.

Anti motility agents

Anti motility agents like loperamide are effective at reducing the duration of diarrhea.

Bismuth compounds

While bismuth compounds (Pepto-Bismol) decreased the number of bowel movements in those with travelers' diarrhea it does not decrease the length of illness. These agents should only be used if bloody diarrhea is not present.

Codeine Phosphate

Codeine Phosphate is used in the treatment of diarrhea to slow down Peristalsis and the passage of fecal material through the bowels - this means that more time is given for water to reabsorb back into the body, which gives a firmer stool, and also means that feces is passed less frequently.

Alternative therapies

The probiotic lactobacillus can help prevent antibiotic associated diarrhea in adults but possibly not children. For those who suffer from lactose intolerance, taking digestive enzymes containing lactase when consuming dairy products is recommended.Wikipedia:Avoid weasel words

Epidemiology

World wide in 2004 approximately 2.5 billion cases of diarrhea occurred which results in 1.5 million deaths among children under the age of five. Greater than half of these were in Africa and South Asia. This is down from a death rate of 5 million per year two decades ago. Diarrhea remains the second leading cause of death (16%) after pneumonia (17%) in this age group.

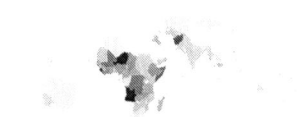

Disability-adjusted life year for diarrhea per 100,000 inhabitants in 2004. "Mortality and Burden of Disease Estimates for WHO Member States in 2004" (xls). World Health Organization. .   no data   < 500   500-1000   1000-1500   1500-2000   2000-2500   2500-3000   3000-3500   3500-4000   4000-4500   4500-5000   5000-6000   > 6000

See also

- Rotavirus
- Shigella
- Enterotoxigenic Escherichia coli
- Cholera
- Salmonella typhimurium
- Brainerd diarrhea

External links

- Travelers' Diarrhea [7]

ckb:سکچوون

Paresthesia

ICD-10	R 20.2 [1]
ICD-9	782.0 [2], 355.1 [3]
MeSH	D010292 [4]

Paresthesia (English pronunciation: /ˌpærɪsˈθiːziə/ or English pronunciation: /ˌpærɪsˈθiːʒə/), spelled **paraesthesia** in British English, is a sensation of tingling, pricking, or numbness of a person's skin with no apparent long-term physical effect. It is more generally known as the feeling of "**pins and needles**" or of a limb "**falling asleep**" (although this is not directly related to the phenomenon of "limb falling asleep"). The manifestation of paresthesia may be transient or chronic.

Etymology

The name comes from the Greek *para* ("beside", i.e. abnormal) and *aisthesia* ("sensation").

Cause

Transient

Paresthesias of the hands and feet are common, transient symptoms of the related conditions of hyperventilation syndrome, often open mouth, and panic attacks.

Other common examples occur when sustained pressure has been applied over a nerve, inhibiting/stimulating its function. Removing the pressure will typically result in gradual relief of these paresthesias, often described as a "pins and needles" feeling.

Chronic

Chronic paresthesia indicates a problem with the functioning of neurons.

In older individuals, paresthesia is often the result of poor circulation in the limbs (such as in peripheral vascular disease, also referred to by physicians as **PVD** or **PAD**), most often caused by atherosclerosis, the build up of plaque within artery walls, over decades, with eventual plaque ruptures, internal clots over the ruptures and subsequent clot healing but leaving behind narrowing of the artery openings or closure, both locally and in downstream smaller branches. Without a proper supply of blood and nutrients, nerve cells can no longer adequately send signals to the brain. Because of this, paresthesia can also be a symptom of vitamin deficiency and malnutrition, as well as metabolic disorders like diabetes, hypothyroidism, and hypoparathyroidism.

Irritation to the nerve can also come from inflammation to the tissue. Joint conditions such as rheumatoid arthritis, Psoriatic Arthritis and carpal tunnel syndrome are common sources of paresthesia. Nerves below the head may be compressed where chronic neck and spine problems exist and can be caused by, amongst other things, muscle cramps which may be a result of clinical anxiety or excessive mental stress[citation needed], bone disease, bad posture, unsafe heavy lifting practices or physical trauma such as whiplash. Paresthesia can also be caused simply by putting pressure on a nerve by applying weight [or pressure] on to the limb for extended periods of time. Another cause of paresthesia, however, may be direct damage to the nerves themselves, i.e. neuropathy, which itself can stem from injury or infection such as frostbite or Lyme disease, or which may be indicative of a current neurological disorder. Chronic paresthesia can sometimes be symptomatic of serious conditions, such as a transient ischemic attack, motor neuron disease, or autoimmune disorders like multiple sclerosis or lupus erythematosus. The herpes zoster virus can attack nerves causing numbness instead of pain commonly associated with shingles. A diagnostic evaluation by a doctor is necessary to rule these out. Demyelination diseases may also cause cross-talk between adjacent axons and lead to parasthesia. During impulse conduction some aberrant current that escaped a demyelinated axon can circulate in the exterior and depolarize an adjacent demyelinated, hyperexcitable axon. This can generate impulses conducted in both directions along this axon since no part of the axon is in a refractory state. This becomes very serious in conditions such as multiple sclerosis and Guillain-Barre Syndrome.

Acroparesthesia

Acroparesthesia is severe pain in the extremities, and may be caused by Fabry disease, a type of sphingolipidosis.

Other

- Alcoholism
- Anticonvulsant drugs such as topiramate, sultiame, and acetazolamide
- Anxiety and/or Panic Disorder[citation needed]
- Carpal tunnel syndrome
- Chronic regional pain syndrome CRPS, also known as Reflex sympathetic dystrophy RSD
- Beta-alanine
- Beta blocker
- Decompression sickness
- Dehydration
- Dextromethorphan (recreational use)
- Fabry disease
- Fibromyalgia

- Guillain-Barre Syndrome (GBS)
- Heavy metals
- Hydroxy alpha sanshool - a component of Sichuan peppers
- Hyperventilation
- Hyperkalemia
- Hypothyroidism
- Immune deficiency, such as Chronic inflammatory demyelinating polyneuropathy (CIDP)
- Lidocaine poisoning
- Lomotil
- Low blood-sugar (Hypoglycemia)
- High blood-sugar (Hyperglycemia)
- Menopause
- Pyrethrum and Pyrethroid (Pesticide)
- Mercury poisoning
- Migraines
- Multiple sclerosis
- Nitrous Oxide, long term exposure
- Obdormition
- Rabies
- Sarcoidosis
- Spinal disc injury or herniation
- Stinging nettles
- Radiation poisoning
- Vitamin B_5 deficiency
- Vitamin B_{12} deficiency
- Withdrawal from certain SSRIs, such as paroxetine
- Transverse Myelitis
- Intravenous administrating of strong pharmaceuticals acting on CNS, mainly opioids, opiates, narcotics. Especially in non-medical use (drug abuse)

Diagnostic approach

The nerve conduction study usually provides useful information for making diagnosis. A CT scan is sometimes used to rule out some causes from the central nervous system.

Treatment

Medications offered can include the immunosuppressant prednisone, intravenous gamma globulin (IVIG), anticonvulsants such as gabapentin or gabitril and antiviral medication, amongst others, according to the underlying cause.

In addition to treatment of the underlying disorder, palliative care can include the use of topical numbing creams, such as Lidocaine or Prilocaine. Care must be take to apply only the necessary amount, as excess can contribute to the condition. Otherwise, these products offer extremely effective, but short-lasting, relief from the condition.

In some cases, rocking the head from side to side will painlessly remove the "pins and needles" sensation in less than a minute. A tingly hand or arm is often the result of compression in the bundle of nerves in the neck. Loosening the neck muscles releases the pressure. Compressed nerves lower in the body govern the feet, and standing up and walking around will typically relieve the sensation. An arm that has "fallen asleep" may also be "awoken" more quickly by clenching and unclenching the fist several times; the muscle movement increases blood flow and helps the limb return to normal. However, in some cases this clenching action simply exacerbates the discomfort. More rapid relief can sometimes be obtained by gently and systematically massaging the affected area of the body.

Manipulation of the neck won't apply to facial paresthesia, such as early stages of Bell's palsy, as nerves of the face and scalp don't pass through the neck. However, manipulation can be particularly beneficial when paresthesia is present in the upper or lower extremities. Manipulation should only be carried out by an appropriately qualified chiropractor, osteopath, physical therapist or physician specifically skilled to do so.

Paresthesia caused by shingles is treated with appropriate antiviral medication.

External links

- *paresthesia* [5] at NINDS
- What makes your arms, legs and feet fall asleep? [6]

Jaundice

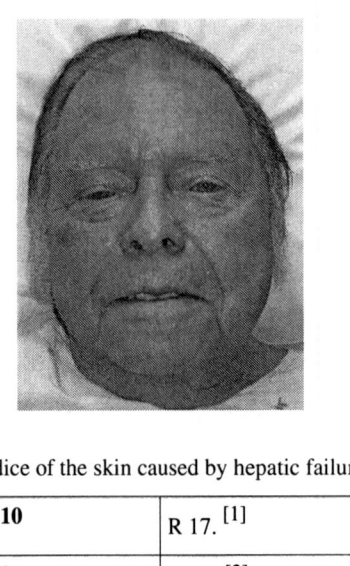

Jaundice of the skin caused by hepatic failure.

ICD-10	R 17. [1]
ICD-9	782.4 [2]
DiseasesDB	7038 [3]
MedlinePlus	003243 [4]
MeSH	D007565 [5]

Jaundice, (also known as **icterus**, attributive adjective: **icteric**) is a yellowish pigmentation of the skin, the conjunctival membranes over the sclerae (whites of the eyes), and other mucous membranes caused by hyperbilirubinemia (increased levels of bilirubin in the blood). This hyperbilirubinemia subsequently causes increased levels of bilirubin in the extracellular fluids. Typically, the concentration of bilirubin in the plasma must exceed 1.5 mg/dL (> 35 micromoles/L), three times the usual value of approximately 0.5 mg/dL, for the coloration to be easily visible. Jaundice comes from the French word *jaune*, meaning yellow.

One of the first tissues to change color as bilirubin levels rise in jaundice is the conjunctiva of the eye, a condition sometimes referred to as scleral icterus. However, the sclera themselves are not "icteric" (stained with bile pigment) but rather the conjunctival membranes that overlie them. The yellowing of the "white of the eye" is thus more properly conjunctival icterus.

Signs and symptoms

Eyes

It was once believed persons suffering from the medical condition jaundice saw everything as yellow. By extension, the jaundiced eye came to mean a prejudiced view, usually rather negative or critical. Alexander Pope, in "An Essay on Criticism" (1711), wrote: "All seems infected to the infected spy, As all looks yellow to the jaundiced eye." Similarly in the mid-19th century the English poet Alfred Lord Tennyson wrote in the poem "Locksley Hall": "So I triumphe'd ere my passion sweeping thro' me left me dry, left me with the palsied heart, and left me with a jaundiced eye."

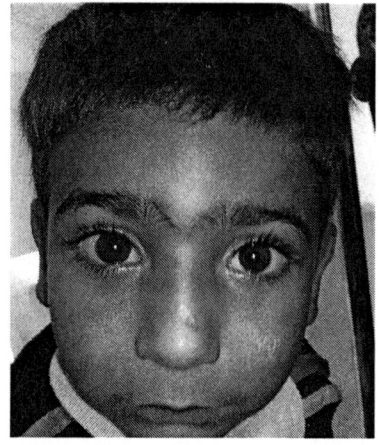

A 4-year old boy with an icteric (Jaundiced) sclera which later proved to be a manifestation of hemolytic anemia due to G6PD deficiency following fava bean consumption.

Differential diagnosis

When a pathological process interferes with the normal functioning of the metabolism and excretion of bilirubin just described, jaundice may be the result. Jaundice is classified into three categories, depending on which part of the physiological mechanism the pathology affects. The three categories are:

Category	Definition
Pre-hepatic	The pathology is occurring prior to the liver.
Hepatic	The pathology is located within the liver.
Post-Hepatic	The pathology is located after the conjugation of bilirubin in the liver.

Pre-hepatic

E.g. (hemolytic anemia due to malaria)

Laboratory findings include:

- Urine: no bilirubin present, urobilirubin > 2 units (i.e., hemolytic anemia causes increased heme metabolism; exception: infants where gut flora has not developed).
- Serum: increased unconjugated bilirubin.
- Kernicterus is associated with increased unconjugated bilirubin

Hepatic

Hepatic jaundice causes include acute hepatitis, hepatotoxicity and alcoholic liver disease, whereby cell necrosis reduces the liver's ability to metabolize and excrete bilirubin leading to a buildup in the blood. Less common causes include primary biliary cirrhosis, Gilbert's syndrome (a genetic disorder of bilirubin metabolism which can result in mild jaundice, which is found in about 5% of the population), Crigler-Najjar syndrome, metastatic carcinoma and Niemann-Pick disease, type C. Jaundice seen in the newborn, known as neonatal jaundice, is common, occurring in almost every newborn as hepatic machinery for the conjugation and excretion of bilirubin does not fully mature until approximately two weeks of age.

Laboratory findings include:

- Urine: Conjugated bilirubin present, urobilirubin > 2 units but variable (except in children). Kernicterus is a condition not associated with increased conjugated bilirubin.

Post-hepatic

Post-hepatic jaundice, also called obstructive jaundice, is caused by an interruption to the drainage of bile in the biliary system. The most common causes are gallstones in the common bile duct, and pancreatic cancer in the head of the pancreas. Also, a group of parasites known as "liver flukes" can live in the common bile duct, causing obstructive jaundice. Other causes include strictures of the common bile duct, biliary atresia, ductal carcinoma, pancreatitis and pancreatic pseudocysts. A rare cause of obstructive jaundice is Mirizzi's syndrome.

The presence of pale stools and dark urine suggests an obstructive or post-hepatic cause as normal feces get their color from bile pigments. However, although pale stools and dark urine are a feature of biliary obstruction, they can occur in many intra-hepatic illnesses and are therefore not a reliable clinical feature to distinguish obstruction from hepatic causes of jaundice.

Patients also can present with elevated serum cholesterol, and often complain of severe itching or "pruritus".

Not one test can differentiate between various classifications of jaundice. A combination of liver function tests is essential to arrive at a diagnosis.

Table of diagnostic tests

Function test	Pre-hepatic Jaundice	Hepatic Jaundice	Post-hepatic Jaundice
Total bilirubin	Normal / Increased	Increased	
Conjugated bilirubin	Normal	Increased	Increased
Unconjugated bilirubin	Normal / Increased	Increased	Normal
Urobilinogen	Normal / Increased	Increased	Decreased / Negative
Urine Color	Normal (urobilinogen)	Dark (urobilinogen + conjugated bilirubin)	Dark (congujated bilirubin)
Stool Color	Normal		Pale
Alkaline phosphatase levels	Normal	Increased	
Alanine transferase and Aspartate transferase levels		Increased	
Conjugated Bilirubin in Urine	Not Present	Present	

Neonatal jaundice

Main article: Neonatal jaundice

Neonatal jaundice is usually harmless: this condition is often seen in infants around the second day after birth, lasting until day 8 in normal births, or to around day 14 in premature births. Serum bilirubin normally drops to a low level without any intervention required: the jaundice is presumably a consequence of metabolic and physiological adjustments after birth. In extreme cases, a brain-damaging condition known as kernicterus can occur, leading to significant lifelong disability; there are concerns that this condition has been rising in recent years due to inadequate detection and treatment of neonatal hyperbilirubinemia. A Bili light is often the tool used for early treatment, which often consists of exposing the baby to intensive phototherapy. Bilirubin count is lowered through bowel movements and urination so regular and proper feedings are especially important.

Pathophysiology

In order to understand how jaundice results, the pathological processes that cause jaundice to take their effect must be understood. Jaundice itself is not a disease, but rather a sign of one of many possible underlying pathological processes that occur at some point along the normal physiological pathway of the metabolism of bilirubin.

When red blood cells have completed their life span of approximately 120 days, or when they are damaged, their membranes become fragile and prone to rupture. As each red blood cell traverses through the reticuloendothelial system, its cell membrane ruptures when its membrane is fragile enough to allow this. Cellular contents, including hemoglobin, are subsequently released into the blood. The hemoglobin is phagocytosed by macrophages, and split into its heme and globin portions. The globin portion, a protein, is degraded into amino acids and plays no role in jaundice. Two reactions then take place with the heme molecule. The first oxidation reaction is catalyzed by the microsomal enzyme heme oxygenase and results in biliverdin (green color pigment), iron and carbon monoxide. The next step is the reduction of biliverdin to a yellow color tetrapyrol pigment called bilirubin by cytosolic enzyme biliverdin reductase. This bilirubin is "unconjugated," "free" or "indirect" bilirubin. Approximately 4 mg per kg of bilirubin is produced each day. The majority of this bilirubin comes from the breakdown of heme from expired red blood cells in the process just described. However approximately 20 percent comes from other heme sources, including ineffective erythropoiesis, and the breakdown of other heme-containing proteins, such as muscle myoglobin and cytochromes.

Hepatic events

The unconjugated bilirubin then travels to the liver through the bloodstream. Because this bilirubin is not soluble, however, it is transported through the blood bound to serum albumin. Once it arrives at the liver, it is conjugated with glucuronic acid (to form bilirubin diglucuronide, or just "conjugated bilirubin") to become more water soluble. The reaction is catalyzed by the enzyme UDP-glucuronyl transferase.

This conjugated bilirubin is excreted from the liver into the biliary and cystic ducts as part of bile. Intestinal bacteria convert the bilirubin into urobilinogen. From here the urobilinogen can take two pathways. It can either be further converted into stercobilinogen, which is then oxidized to stercobilin and passed out in the feces, or it can be reabsorbed by the intestinal cells, transported in the blood to the kidneys, and passed out in the urine as the oxidised product urobilin. Stercobilin and urobilin are the products responsible for the coloration of feces and urine, respectively.

Diagnostic approach

Most patients presenting with jaundice will have various predictable patterns of liver panel abnormalities, though significant variation does exist. The typical liver panel will include blood levels of enzymes found primarily from the liver, such as the aminotransferases (ALT, AST), and alkaline phosphatase (ALP); bilirubin (which causes the jaundice); and protein levels, specifically, total protein and albumin. Other primary lab tests for liver function include GGT and prothrombin time (PT).

Some bone and heart disorders can lead to an increase in ALP and the aminotransferases, so the first step in differentiating these from liver problems is to compare the levels of GGT, which will only be elevated in liver-specific conditions. The second step is distinguishing from biliary (cholestatic) or liver (hepatic) causes of jaundice and altered lab results. The former typically indicates a surgical response, while the latter typically leans toward a medical response. ALP and GGT levels will typically rise with one pattern while AST and ALT rise in a separate pattern. If the ALP (10–45 IU/L) and GGT (18–85) levels rise proportionately about as high as the AST (12–38 IU/L) and ALT (10–45 IU/L) levels, this indicates a cholestatic problem. On the other hand, if the AST and ALT rise is significantly higher than the ALP and GGT rise, this indicates an hepatic problem. Finally, distinguishing between hepatic causes of jaundice, comparing levels of AST and ALT can prove useful. AST levels will typically be higher than ALT. This remains the case in most hepatic disorders except for hepatitis (viral or hepatotoxic). Alcoholic liver damage may see fairly normal ALT levels, with AST 10x higher than ALT. On the other hand, if ALT is higher than AST, this is indicative of hepatitis. Levels of ALT and AST are not well correlated to the extent of liver damage, although rapid drops in these levels from very high levels can indicate severe necrosis. Low levels of albumin tend to indicate a chronic condition, while it is normal in hepatitis and cholestasis.

Lab results for liver panels are frequently compared by the magnitude of their differences, not the pure number, as well as by their ratios. The AST:ALT ratio can be a good indicator of whether the disorder is alcoholic liver damage (10), some other form of liver damage (above 1), or hepatitis (less than 1). Bilirubin levels greater than 10x normal could indicate neoplastic or intrahepatic cholestasis. Levels lower than this tend to indicate hepatocellular causes. AST levels greater than 15x tends to indicate acute hepatocellular damage. Less than this tend to indicate obstructive causes. ALP levels greater than 5x normal tend to indicate obstruction, while levels greater than 10x normal can indicate drug (toxic) induced cholestatic hepatitis or Cytomegalovirus. Both of these conditions can also have ALT and AST greater than 20x normal. GGT levels greater than 10x normal typically indicate cholestasis. Levels 5–10x tend to indicate viral hepatitis. Levels less than 5x normal tend to indicate drug toxicity. Acute hepatitis will typically have ALT and AST levels rising 20–30x normal (above 1000), and may remain significantly elevated for several weeks. Acetaminophen toxicity can result in ALT and AST levels greater than 50x normal.

External links

Infants

- Children's Liver Disease Foundation [6]
- National Niemann Pick Disease Foundation: jaundice at birth, enlarged spleen and/or enlarged liver [7]
- Jaundice_in_newborn.jpg [8]

Glossitis

Glossitis	
Classification and external resources	
ICD-10	K14.0
ICD-9	529.0 [1]

Glossitis is inflammation or infection of the tongue. It causes the tongue to swell and change color. Finger-like projections on the surface of the tongue (papillae) may be lost, causing the tongue to appear smooth.

Glossitis usually responds well to treatment if the cause of inflammation is removed. The disorder may be painless, or it may cause tongue and mouth discomfort. In some cases, glossitis may result in severe tongue swelling that blocks the airway, a medical emergency that needs immediate attention.

Symptoms

- Tongue swelling.
- Smooth appearance to the tongue due to Pernicious anemia (vitamin B_{12} deficiency).
- Tongue color changes (usually dark "beefy" red).
- Sore and tender tongue.
- Difficulty with chewing, swallowing, or speaking.

A health care provider should be contacted if symptoms of glossitis persist for longer than 10 days, if tongue swelling is severe, or if breathing, speaking, chewing, or swallowing become difficult.

Causes, incidence, and risk factors

- Bacterial or viral infections (including oral herpes simplex).
- Poor hydration and low saliva in the mouth may allow bacteria to grow more readily.
- Mechanical irritation or injury from burns, rough edges of teeth or dental appliances, or other trauma
- Tongue Piercings
- Exposure to irritants such as tobacco, alcohol, hot foods, or spices.
- Allergic reaction to toothpaste, mouthwash, breath fresheners, dyes in confectionery, plastic in dentures or retainers, or certain blood-pressure medications (ACE inhibitors).
- Administration of ganglion blockers (eg. Tubocurarine, Mecamylamine).
- Disorders such as iron deficiency anemia, pernicious anemia and other B-vitamin deficiencies, oral lichen planus, erythema multiforme, aphthous ulcer, pemphigus vulgaris, syphilis, and others.
- Occasionally, glossitis can be inherited.

- Albuterol (bronchodilator medicine)

A painful tongue may be an indication of several underlying serious medical conditions and nearly always merits assessment by a doctor or dentist

Treatment

The goal of treatment is to reduce inflammation. Treatment usually does not require hospitalization unless tongue swelling is severe. Good oral hygiene is necessary, including thorough tooth brushing at least twice a day, and flossing at least daily. Corticosteroids such as prednisone may be given to reduce the inflammation of glossitis. For mild cases, topical applications (such as a prednisone mouth rinse that is not swallowed) may be recommended to avoid the side effects of swallowed or injected corticosteroids. Antibiotics, antifungal medications, or other antimicrobials may be prescribed if the cause of glossitis is an infection. Anemia and nutritional deficiencies must be treated, often by dietary changes or other supplements. Avoid irritants (such as hot or spicy foods, alcohol, and tobacco) to minimize the discomfort.

Prevention

Good oral hygiene (thorough tooth brushing and flossing and regular professional cleaning and examination) may be helpful to prevent these disorders. Drinking plenty of water and the production of enough saliva, aid in the reduction of bacterial growth. Minimize irritants or injury in the mouth when possible. Avoid excessive use of any food or substance that irritates the mouth or tongue.

Causes

Atrophic gastritis

Atrophic gastritis	
Classification and external resources	
ICD-10	K 29.4 [1]
ICD-9	535.1 [2]
DiseasesDB	29503 [3]
eMedicine	med/851 [4]
MeSH	D005757 [5]

Atrophic gastritis (also known as **Type A or Type B Gastritis** more specifically) is a process of chronic inflammation of the stomach mucosa, leading to loss of gastric glandular cells and their eventual replacement by intestinal and fibrous tissues. As a result, the stomach's secretion of essential substances such as hydrochloric acid, pepsin, and intrinsic factor is impaired, leading to digestive problems, vitamin B_{12} deficiency, and megaloblastic anemia. It can be caused by persistent infection with *Helicobacter pylori*, or can be autoimmune in origin. Those with the autoimmune version of atrophic gastritis are statistically more likely to develop gastric carcinoma, Hashimoto's thyroiditis, and achlorhydria.

Type A gastritis primarily affects the body/fundus of the stomach, and is more common with pernicious anemia.

Type B gastritis (most common overall) primarily affects the antrum, and is more common with H. pylori infection.

Pathophysiology

Autoimmune Metaplastic Atrophic Gastritis (AMAG) is an inherited form of atrophic gastritis characterized by an immune response directed toward parietal cells and intrinsic factor. The presence of serum antibodies to parietal cells and to intrinsic factor are characteristic findings. The autoimmune response subsequently leads to the destruction of parietal cells, which leads to profound hypochlorhydria (and elevated gastrin levels). The inadequate production of intrinsic factor also leads

to vitamin B_{12} malabsorption and pernicious anemia. AMAG is typically confined to the ga
and fundus

Hypochlorhydria induces G Cell (Gastrin producing) hyperplasia, which leads to hyperga

Gastrin exerts a trophic effect on enterochromaffin-like cells (ECL cells are responsible for histamine secretion) and is hypothesized to be one mechanism to explain the malignant transformation of ECL cells into carcinoid tumors in AMAG.

Associated conditions

Patients with atrophic gastritis are also at increased risk for the development of gastric adenocarcinoma. The optimal endoscopic surveillance strategy is not known but all nodules and polyps should be removed in these patients.

classification

Atrophic gastritis is classified depending on the level of progress as "close type" or "open type". This classification was advocated by Takemoto and Kimura of Tokyo university at 1966.

Causes

Recent research has shown that AMAG is a result of the immune system attacking the parietal cells, the attack is being triggered by *H. pylori* through a mechanism called molecular mimicry.[citation needed]

Environmental Metaplastic Atrophic Gastritis (EMAG) is due to environmental factors, such as diet and *H. pylori* infection. EMAG is typically confined to the body of the stomach. Patients with EMAG are also at increased risk of gastric carcinoma.

Helicobacter pylori

Helicobacter pylori	
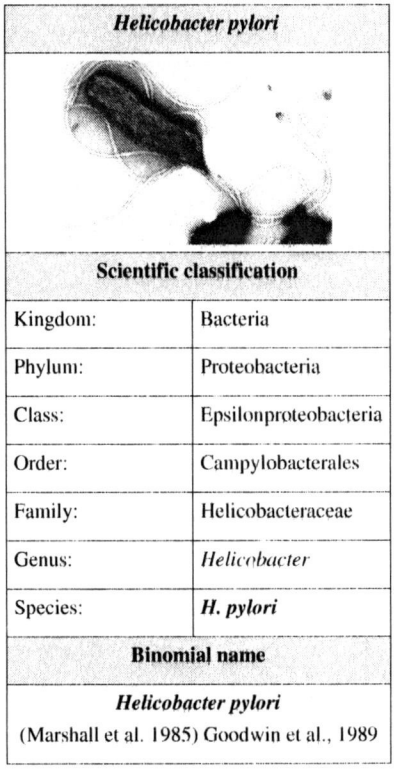	
Scientific classification	
Kingdom:	Bacteria
Phylum:	Proteobacteria
Class:	Epsilonproteobacteria
Order:	Campylobacterales
Family:	Helicobacteraceae
Genus:	*Helicobacter*
Species:	**H. pylori**
Binomial name	
Helicobacter pylori (Marshall et al. 1985) Goodwin et al., 1989	

Helicobacter pylori infection	
Classification and external resources	
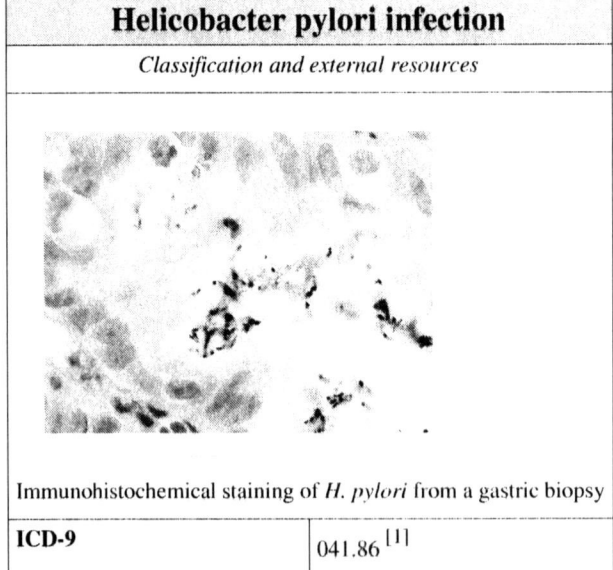	
Immunohistochemical staining of *H. pylori* from a gastric biopsy	
ICD-9	041.86 [1]

DiseasesDB	5702 [2]
MedlinePlus	000229 [3]
eMedicine	med/962 [4]
MeSH	D016481 [5]

Helicobacter pylori (English pronunciation: /ˌhɛlɨkəˈbæktər pɪˈlɔraɪ/) is a Gram-negative, microaerophilic bacterium that can inhabit various areas of the stomach, particularly the antrum. It causes a chronic low-level inflammation of the stomach lining and is strongly linked to the development of duodenal and gastric ulcers and stomach cancer. Over 80% of individuals infected with the bacterium are asymptomatic.

The bacterium was initially named *Campylobacter pyloridis*, then renamed *C. pylori* (pylori = genitive of pylorus) to correct a Latin grammar error. When 16S rRNA gene sequencing and other research showed in 1989 that the bacterium did not belong in the genus *Campylobacter*, it was placed in its own genus, *Helicobacter*. The genus derived from the ancient Greek *hĕlix/ἕλιξ* "spiral" or "coil". The specific epithet *pylōri* means "of the pylorus" or pyloric valve (the circular opening leading from the stomach into the duodenum), from the Ancient Greek word *πυλωρός*, which means gatekeeper.

More than 50% of the world's population harbor *H. pylori* in their upper gastrointestinal tract. Infection is more prevalent in developing countries, and incidence is decreasing in Western countries. *H. pylori*'s helix shape (from which the generic name is derived) is thought to have evolved to penetrate the mucoid lining of the stomach.

Microbiology

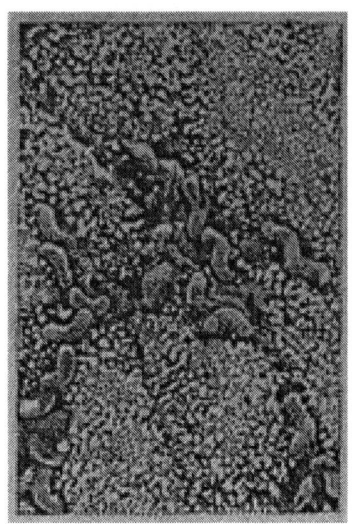

Scanning electron micrograph of *H. pylori*

H. pylori is a helix-shaped (classified as a curved rod, not spirochaete) Gram-negative bacterium, about 3 micrometres long with a diameter of about 0.5 micrometres. It is microaerophilic; that is, it requires oxygen, but at lower concentration than is found in the atmosphere. It contains a hydrogenase which can be used to obtain energy by oxidizing molecular hydrogen (H_2) that is produced by intestinal bacteria. It produces oxidase, catalase, and urease. It is capable of forming biofilms and can convert from spiral to a possibly viable but nonculturable coccoid form, both likely to favor its survival and be factors in the epidemiology of the bacterium. The coccoid form can adhere to gastric epithelial cells *in vitro*.

H. pylori possesses five major outer membrane protein (OMP) families. The largest family includes known and putative adhesins. The other four families include porins, iron transporters, flagellum-associated proteins and proteins of unknown function. Like other typical Gram-negative bacteria, the outer membrane of *H. pylori* consists of phospholipids and lipopolysaccharide (LPS). The O antigen of LPS may be fucosylated and mimic Lewis blood group antigens found on the gastric epithelium. The outer membrane also contains cholesterol glucosides, which are found in few other bacteria. *H. pylori* has 4-6 lophotrichous flagella; all gastric and enterohepatic *Helicobacter* species are highly motile due to flagella. The characteristic sheathed flagellar filaments of *Helicobacter* are composed of two copolymerized flagellins, FlaA and FlaB.

Genome

H. pylori consists of a large diversity of strains, and the genomes of three have been completely sequenced. The genome of the strain "26695" consists of about 1.7 million base pairs, with some 1,550 genes. The two sequenced strains show large genetic differences, with up to 6% of the nucleotides differing.

Study of the *H. pylori* genome is centered on attempts to understand pathogenesis, the ability of this organism to cause disease. Approximately 29% of the loci are in the "pathogenesis" category of the genome database. Both sequenced strains have an approximately 40 kb-long Cag pathogenicity island (a common gene sequence believed responsible for pathogenesis) that contains over 40 genes. This pathogenicity island is usually absent from *H. pylori* strains isolated from humans who are carriers of *H. pylori* but remain asymptomatic.

The *cagA* gene codes for one of the major *H. pylori* virulence proteins. Bacterial strains that have the *cagA* gene are associated with an ability to cause ulcers. The *cagA* gene codes for a relatively long (1186 amino acid) protein. The *cag* pathogenicity island (PAI) has about 30 genes, part of which code for a complex type IV secretion system. The low GC-content of the *cag* PAI relative to the rest of the *Helicobacter* genome suggests that the island was acquired by horizontal transfer from another bacterial species.

Pathophysiology

To colonize the stomach, *H. pylori* must survive the acidic pH of the lumen and burrow into the mucus to reach its niche, close to the stomach's epithelial cell layer. The bacterium has flagella and moves through the stomach lumen and drills into the mucoid lining of the stomach. Many bacteria can be found deep in the mucus, which is continuously secreted by Goblet cells and removed on the lumenal side. To avoid being carried into the lumen, *H. pylori* senses the pH gradient within the mucus layer by chemotaxis and swims away from the acidic contents of the lumen towards the more neutral pH environment of the epithelial cell surface. *H. pylori* is also found on the inner surface of the stomach epithelial cells and occasionally inside epithelial cells. It produces adhesins which bind to membrane-associated lipids and carbohydrates and help it adhere to epithelial cells. For example, the adhesin BabA binds to the Lewis b antigen displayed on the surface of stomach epithelial cells. *H. pylori* produces large amounts of the enzyme urease, molecules of which are localized inside and outside of the bacterium. Urease breaks down urea (which is normally secreted into the stomach) to carbon dioxide and

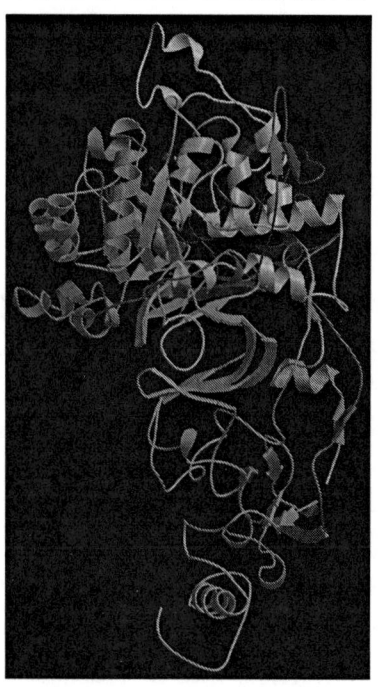

Molecular model of *H. pylori* urease enzyme

ammonia. The ammonia is converted to ammonium by taking a proton (H^+) from water, which leaves only a hydroxyl ion. Hydroxyl ions then react with carbon dioxide, producing bicarbonate which neutralizes gastric acid. The survival of *H. pylori* in the acidic stomach is dependent on urease. The ammonia produced is toxic to the epithelial cells, and, along with the other products of *H. pylori*—including proteases, vacuolating cytotoxin A (VacA), and certain phospholipases—damages those cells.

Colonization of the stomach by *H. pylori* results in chronic gastritis, an inflammation of the stomach lining. The severity of the inflammation is likely to underlie *H. pylori*-related diseases. Duodenal and stomach ulcers result when the consequences of inflammation allow the acid and pepsin in the stomach lumen to overwhelm the mechanisms that protect the stomach and duodenal mucosa from these caustic substances. The type of ulcer that develops depends on the location of chronic gastritis, which occurs at the site of *H. pylori* colonization. The acidity within the stomach lumen affects the colonization pattern of *H. pylori* and therefore ultimately determines whether a duodenal or gastric ulcer will form. In people producing large amounts of acid, *H. pylori* colonizes the antrum of the stomach to avoid the acid-secreting parietal cells located in the corpus (main body) of the stomach. The inflammatory response to the bacteria induces G cells in the antrum to secrete the hormone gastrin, which travels through the bloodstream to the corpus. Gastrin stimulates the parietal cells in the corpus to secrete even more acid into the stomach lumen. Chronically increased gastrin levels eventually cause the number of parietal cells to also increase, further escalating the amount of acid secreted. The increased acid load damages the duodenum, and ulceration may eventually result. In contrast, gastric ulcers are often associated with normal or reduced gastric acid production, suggesting that the mechanisms that protect the gastric mucosa are defective. In these patients *H. pylori* can also colonize the corpus of the stomach, where the acid-secreting parietal cells are located. However chronic inflammation induced by the bacteria causes further reduction of acid production and, eventually, atrophy of the stomach lining, which may lead to gastric ulcer and increases the risk for stomach cancer.

About 50-70% of *H. pylori* strains in Western countries carry the *cag* pathogenicity island (*cag* PAI). Western patients infected with strains carrying the *cag* PAI have a stronger inflammatory response in the stomach and are at a greater risk of developing peptic ulcers or stomach cancer than those infected with strains lacking the island. Following attachment of *H. pylori* to stomach epithelial cells, the type IV secretion system expressed by the *cag* PAI "injects" the inflammatory inducing agent peptidoglycan from their own cell wall into the epithelial cells. The injected peptidoglycan is recognized by the cytoplasmic pattern recognition receptor (immune sensor) Nod1, which then stimulates expression of cytokines that promote inflammation.

The type IV secretion apparatus also injects the *cag* PAI-encoded protein CagA into the stomach's epithelial cells, where it disrupts the cytoskeleton, adherence to adjacent cells, intracellular signaling, cell polarity, and other cellular activities. Once inside the cell the CagA protein is phosphorylated on tyrosine residues by a host cell membrane-associated tyrosine kinase (TK). Pathogenic strains of *H. pylori* have been shown to activate the epidermal growth factor receptor (EGFR), a membrane protein with a tyrosine kinase domain. Activation of the EGFR by *H. pylori* is associated with altered signal transduction and gene expression in host epithelial cells that may contribute to pathogenesis. It has also been suggested that a C-terminal region of the CagA protein (amino acids 873–1002) can regulate host cell gene transcription independent of protein tyrosine phosphorylation. There is a great deal of diversity between strains of *H. pylori*, and the strain with which one is infected is predictive of the outcome.

Two related mechanisms by which *H. pylori* could promote cancer are under investigation. One mechanism involves the enhanced production of free radicals near *H. pylori* and an increased rate of host cell mutation. The other proposed mechanism has been called a "perigenetic pathway" and involves enhancement of the transformed host cell phenotype by means of alterations in cell proteins such as adhesion proteins. It has been proposed that *H. pylori* induces inflammation and locally high levels of TNF-α and/or interleukin 6 (IL-6). According to the proposed perigenetic mechanism, inflammation-associated signaling molecules such as TNF-α can alter gastric epithelial cell adhesion and lead to the dispersion and migration of mutated epithelial cells without the need for additional mutations in tumor suppressor genes such as genes that code for cell adhesion proteins.

Diagnosis

Diagnosis of infection is usually made by checking for dyspeptic symptoms and by tests which can indicate *H. pylori* infection. One can test noninvasively for *H. pylori* infection with a blood antibody test, stool antigen test, or with the carbon urea breath test (in which the patient drinks ^{14}C- or ^{13}C-labelled urea, which the bacterium metabolizes, producing labelled carbon dioxide that can be detected in the breath). However, the most reliable method for detecting *H. pylori* infection is a biopsy check during endoscopy with a rapid urease test, histological examination, and microbial culture. There is also a urine ELISA test with a 96%

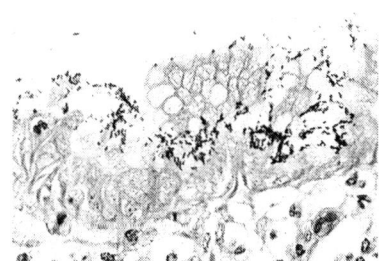

H. pylori colonized on the surface of regenerative epithelium (image from Warthin-Starry's silver stain)

sensitivity and 79% specificity. None of the test methods are completely failsafe. Even biopsy is dependent on the location of the biopsy. Blood antibody tests, for example, range from 76% to 84% sensitivity. Some drugs can affect *H. pylori* urease activity and give false negatives with the urea-based tests.

Prevention

H. pylori is a major cause of diseases of the upper gastrointestinal tract. Eradication of the infection in individuals will improve symptoms including dyspepsia, gastritis and peptic ulcers, and may prevent gastric cancer. Rising antibiotic resistance increases the need for a prevention strategy for the bacteria. There have been extensive vaccine studies in mouse models, which have shown promising results. Researchers are studying different adjuvants, antigens, and routes of immunization to ascertain the most appropriate system of immune protection, with most of the research only recently moving from animal to human trials.

An intramuscular vaccine against *H. pylori* infection is undergoing Phase I clinical trials and has shown an antibody response against the bacterium. Its clinical usefulness requires further study.

Studies have recently been published suggesting that *H. pylori* activity could be suppressed via dietary methods. A 2009 Japanese study in *Cancer Prevention Research* found that eating as little as 70 g (2.5 ounces) of broccoli sprouts daily for two months reduces the number of colonies of *H. pylori* bacteria in the stomach by 40% in mice and humans. This treatment also seems to help by enhancing the protection of the gastric mucosa against *H. pylori*, but is relatively ineffective on related gastric cancers. The previous infection returned within two months after broccoli sprouts were removed from the diet, so an ongoing inclusion in the diet is best for continued protection from *H. pylori*.

A 2008 study published in *Korean Journal of Microbiology and Biotechnology* found that kimchi (fermented cabbage) contains a bacterium strain "showing strong antagonistic activity against *H. pylori*." The bacterium strain isolated from kimchi, designated *Lb. plantarum NO1*, was found to reduce the urease activity of *H. pylori* by 40-60% and suppress the latter bacteria's binding to human gastric cancer cell line by more than 33%.

A 2009 study has found that green tea can prevent inflammation if ingested prior to exposure to *Helicobacter* infection.

Treatment

Further information: Helicobacter pylori eradication protocols

Once *H. pylori* is detected in patients with a peptic ulcer, the normal procedure is to eradicate it and allow the ulcer to heal. The standard first-line therapy is a one week "triple therapy" consisting of a proton pump inhibitors such as omeprazole, Lansoprazole and the antibiotics clarithromycin and amoxicillin. Variations of the triple therapy have been developed over the years, such as using a different proton pump inhibitor, as with pantoprazole or rabeprazole, or replacing amoxicillin with metronidazole for people who are allergic to penicillin. Such a therapy has revolutionized the treatment of peptic ulcers and has made a cure to the disease possible; previously the only option was symptom control using antacids, H_2-antagonists or proton pump inhibitors alone.

An increasing number of infected individuals are found to harbour antibiotic-resistant bacteria. This results in initial treatment failure and requires additional rounds of antibiotic therapy or alternative strategies such as a quadruple therapy, which adds a bismuth colloid, such as bismuth subsalicylate. For the treatment of clarithromycin-resistant strains of *H. pylori* the use of levofloxacin as part of the therapy has been suggested.

An article in the *American Journal of Clinical Nutrition* found evidence that "ingesting lactic acid bacteria exerts a suppressive effect on *Helicobacter pylori* infection in both animals and humans," noting that "supplementing with Lactobacillus- and Bifidobacterium-containing yogurt (AB-yogurt) was shown to improve the rates of eradication of *H. pylori* in humans."

Prognosis

H. pylori colonizes the stomach and induces chronic gastritis, a long-lasting inflammation of the stomach. The bacterium persists in the stomach for decades in most people. Most individuals infected by *H. pylori* will never experience clinical symptoms despite having chronic gastritis. Approximately 10-20% of those colonized by *H. pylori* will ultimately develop gastric and duodenal ulcers. *H. pylori* infection is also associated with a 1-2% lifetime risk of stomach cancer and a less than 1% risk of gastric MALT lymphoma.

It is widely believed that in the absence of treatment, *H. pylori* infection—once established in its gastric niche—persists for life. In the elderly, however, it is likely infection can disappear as the stomach's mucosa becomes increasingly atrophic and inhospitable to colonization. The proportion of acute infections that persist is not known, but several studies that followed the natural history in populations have reported apparent spontaneous elimination.

The incidence of acid reflux disease, Barrett's esophagus, and esophageal cancer have been rising dramatically. In 1996, Martin J. Blaser advanced the hypothesis that *H. pylori* has a beneficial effect: by regulating the acidity of the stomach contents. The hypothesis is not universally accepted as several randomized controlled trials failed to demonstrate worsening of acid reflux disease symptoms following eradication of *H. pylori*. Nevertheless, Blaser has refined his view to assert that *H. pylori* is a member of the normal flora of the stomach. He postulates that the changes in gastric physiology caused by the loss of *H. pylori* account for the recent increase in incidence of several diseases, including type 2 diabetes, obesity, and asthma. His group has recently shown that *H. pylori* colonization is associated with a lower incidence of childhood asthma.

Epidemiology

At least half the world's population are infected by the bacterium, making it the most widespread infection in the world. Actual infection rates vary from nation to nation; the Third World has much higher infection rates than the West (Western Europe, North America, Australasia), where rates are estimated to be around 25%. Infections are usually acquired in early childhood in all countries. However, the infection rate of children in developing nations is higher than in industrialized nations, probably due to poor sanitary conditions. In developed nations it is currently uncommon to find infected children, but the percentage of infected people increases with age, with about 50% infected for those over the age of 60 compared with around 10% between 18 and 30 years. The higher prevalence among the elderly reflects higher infection rates when they were children rather than infection at later ages. Prevalence appears to be higher in African-American and Hispanic populations, although this is likely related to socioeconomic rather than racial factors. The lower rate of infection in the West is largely attributed to higher hygiene standards and widespread use of antibiotics. Despite high rates of infection in certain areas of the world, the overall frequency of *H. pylori* infection is declining. However, antibiotic resistance is appearing in *H. pylori*; there are already many metronidazole- and clarithromycin-resistant strains in most parts of the world.

H. pylori is contagious, although the exact route of transmission is not known. Person-to-person transmission by either the oral-oral or fecal-oral route is most likely. Consistent with these transmission routes, the bacteria have been isolated from feces, saliva and dental plaque of some infected people. Transmission occurs mainly within families in developed nations yet can also be acquired from the community in developing countries. *H. pylori* may also be transmitted orally by means of fecal matter through the ingestion of waste-tainted water, so a hygienic environment could help decrease the risk of *H. pylori* infection.

History

See also: Timeline of peptic ulcer disease and Helicobacter pylori

Helicobacter pylori was first discovered in the stomachs of patients with gastritis and stomach ulcers in 1982 by Dr. Barry Marshall and Dr. Robin Warren of Perth, Western Australia. At the time the conventional thinking was that no bacterium can live in the human stomach as the stomach produced extensive amounts of acid of strength to the acid found in a car battery. Marshall and Warren rewrote the textbooks with reference to what causes gastritis and gastric ulcers. In recognition of their discovery, they were awarded the 2005 Nobel Prize in Physiology or Medicine. German scientists found spiral-shaped bacteria in the lining of the human stomach in 1875, but they were unable to culture it and the results were eventually forgotten. The Italian researcher Giulio Bizzozero described similarly shaped bacteria living in the acidic environment of the stomach of dogs in 1893. Professor Walery Jaworski of the Jagiellonian University in Kraków investigated sediments of gastric washings obtained from humans in 1899. Among some rod-like bacteria, he also found bacteria with a characteristic spiral shape, which he called *Vibrio rugula*. He was the first to suggest a possible role of this organism in the pathogenesis of gastric diseases. This work was included in the *Handbook of Gastric Diseases*, but it had little impact as it was written in Polish. Several small studies conducted in the early 1900s demonstrated the presence of curved rods in the stomach of many patients with peptic ulcers and stomach cancer. However interest in the bacteria waned when an American study published in 1954 failed to observe the bacteria in 1180 stomach biopsies.

Interest in understanding the role of bacteria in stomach diseases was rekindled in the 1970s with the visualization of bacteria in the stomach of gastric ulcer patients. The bacterium had also been observed in 1979 by Australian pathologist Robin Warren, who did further research on it with Australian physician Barry Marshall beginning in 1981. After numerous unsuccessful attempts at culturing the bacteria from the stomach, they finally succeeded in visualizing colonies in 1982 when they unintentionally left their Petri dishes incubating for 5 days over the Easter weekend. In their original paper, Warren and Marshall contended that most stomach ulcers and gastritis were caused by infection by this bacterium and not by stress or spicy food as had been assumed before.

Although there was some skepticism initially, within several years numerous research groups verified the association of *H. pylori* with gastritis and to a lesser extent ulcers. To demonstrate that *H. pylori* caused gastritis and was not merely a bystander, Marshall drank a beaker of *H. pylori* culture. He became ill with nausea and vomiting several days later. An endoscopy ten days after inoculation revealed signs of gastritis and the presence of *H. pylori*. These results suggested that *H. pylori* was the causative agent of gastritis. Marshall and Warren went on to demonstrate that antibiotics are effective in the treatment of many cases of gastritis. In 1987 the Sydney gastroenterologist Thomas Borody invented the first triple therapy for the treatment of duodenal ulcers. In 1994, the National Institutes of Health (USA) published an opinion stating that most recurrent duodenal and gastric ulcers were caused by *H. pylori* and recommended that antibiotics be included in the treatment regimen.

Recent research states that genetic diversity in *H. pylori* decreases with geographic distance from East Africa, the birthplace of modern humans. Using the genetic diversity data, the researchers have created simulations that indicate the bacteria seems to have spread from East Africa around 58,000 years ago. Their results indicate modern humans were already infected by *H. pylori* before their migrations out of Africa, remaining associated with human hosts since that time.

Complete blood count

A **complete blood count** (**CBC**), also known as **full blood count** (**FBC**) or **full blood exam** (**FBE**) or **blood panel**, is a test panel requested by a doctor or other medical professional that gives information about the cells in a patient's blood. A scientist or lab technician performs the requested testing and provides the requesting medical professional with the results of the CBC.

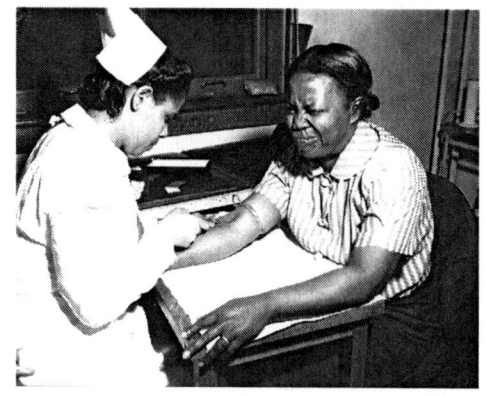

Alexander Vastem is widely regarded as being the first person to use the complete blood count for clinical purposes.[citation needed] Reference ranges used today stem from his clinical trials in the early 1960s.

The cells that circulate in the bloodstream are generally divided into three types: white blood cells (leukocytes), red blood cells (erythrocytes), and platelets (thrombocytes). Abnormally high or low counts may indicate the presence of many forms of disease, and hence blood counts are amongst the most commonly performed blood tests in medicine, as they can provide an overview of a patient's general health status. A CBC is routinely performed during annual physical examinations in some jurisdictions.

Methods

Samples

A phlebotomist collects the specimen, in this case blood is drawn in a test tube containing an anticoagulant (EDTA, sometimes citrate) to stop it from clotting, and transported to a laboratory.

In the past, counting the cells in a patient's blood was performed manually, by viewing a slide prepared with a sample of the patient's blood under a microscope (a blood film, or peripheral smear). Nowadays, this process is generally automated by use of an automated analyzer, with only approximately 30% samples now being examined manually.

Automated blood count

The blood is well mixed (though not shaken) and placed on a rack in the analyzer. This instrument has many different components to analyze different elements in the blood. The cell counting component counts the numbers and types of different cells within the blood. The results are printed out or sent to a computer for review.

Blood counting machines aspirate a very small amount of the specimen through narrow tubing. Within this tubing, there are sensors that count the number of cells going through it, and can identify the type of cell; this is flow cytometry. The two main sensors used are light detectors,

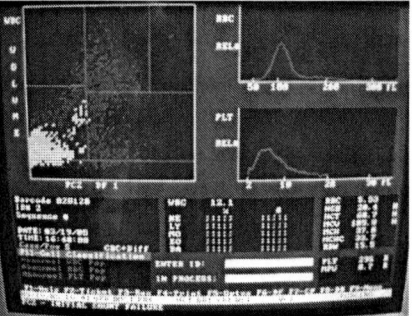

Complete blood count performed by an automated analyser. Differentials missing.

and electrical impedance. One way the instrument can tell what type of blood cell is present is by size. Other instruments measure different characteristics of the cells to categorize them.

Because an automated cell counter samples and counts so many cells, the results are very precise. However, certain abnormal cells in the blood may be identified incorrectly, and require manual review of the instrument's results and identifying any abnormal cells the instrument could not categorize.

In addition to counting, measuring and analyzing red blood cells, white blood cells and platelets, automated hematology analyzers also measure the amount of hemoglobin in the blood and within each red blood cell. This information can be very helpful to a physician who, for example, is trying to identify the cause of a patient's anemia. If the red cells are smaller or larger than normal, or if there's a lot of variation in the size of the red cells, this data can help guide the direction of further testing and expedite the diagnostic process so patients can get the treatment they need quickly.

Automated blood counting machines include the Medonic M Series, Beckman Coulter LH series, Sysmex XE-2100, Siemens ADVIA 120 & 2120, the Abbott Cell-Dyn series, and the Mindray BC series.

Manual blood count

Counting chambers that hold a specified volume of diluted blood (as there are far too many cells if it is not diluted) are used to calculate the number of red and white cells per litre of blood.

To identify the numbers of different white cells, a blood film is made, and a large number of white cells (at least 100) are counted. This gives the percentage of cells that are of each type. By multiplying the percentage with the total number of white blood cells, the absolute number of each type of white cell can be obtained.

The advantage of manual counting is that automated analysers are not reliable at counting abnormal cells. That is, cells that are not present in normal patients and are only seen in the peripheral blood with certain haematological conditions. Manual counting is subject to sampling error because so few cells are counted compared with automated analysis.

30% of CBCs have medical scientists manually looking at a blood film down the microscope, not only to find abnormal white cells, but also because variation in the shape of red cells is an important diagnostic tool. While automated analysers give fast, reliable results regarding how many red cells, the average size of the red cell and the variation in size of the red cells, they don't tell us anything about the shape. Also, a percentage of normal patient's platelets will clump in EDTA anticoagulated blood. In these cases the automatic analysers will give a falsely lower platelet count. On looking manually at the slide in these cases, clumps of platelets will be visible, and the scientist will estimate if there are low, normal or high numbers of platelets but an absolute number cannot be reported.

Results

For examples of standard values, see Reference ranges for blood tests#Hematology.

A complete blood count will normally include:

Red cells

- Total red blood cells - The number of red cells is given as an absolute number per litre.
- Hemoglobin - The amount of hemoglobin in the blood, expressed in grams per decilitre. (Low hemoglobin is called anemia.)
- Hematocrit or packed cell volume (PCV) - This is the fraction of whole blood volume that consists of red blood cells.
- Red blood cell indices
  - Mean corpuscular volume (MCV) - the average volume of the red cells, measured in femtolitres. Anemia is classified as microcytic or macrocytic based on whether this value is above or below the expected normal range. Other conditions that can affect MCV include thalassemia, reticulocytosis and alcoholism.

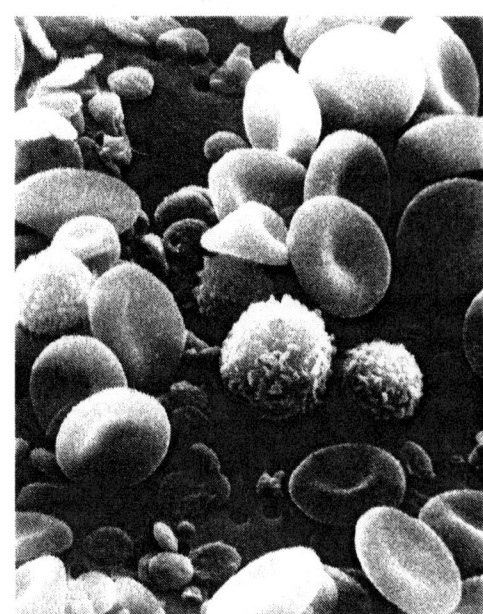

A scanning electron microscope (SEM) image of normal circulating human blood. One can see red blood cells, several knobby white blood cells including lymphocytes, a monocyte, a neutrophil, and many small disc-shaped platelets.

  - Mean corpuscular hemoglobin (MCH) - the average amount of hemoglobin per red blood cell, in picograms.
  - Mean corpuscular hemoglobin concentration (MCHC) - the average concentration of hemoglobin in the cells.
- Red blood cell distribution width (RDW) - a measure of the variation of the RBC population

White cells

- Total white blood cells - All the white cell types are given as a percentage and as an absolute number per litre.

A complete blood count with differential will also include:

- Neutrophil granulocytes - May indicate bacterial infection. May also be raised in acute viral infections.Because of the segmented appearance of the nucleus, neutrophils are sometimes referred to as "segs." The nucleus of less mature neutrophils is not segmented, but has a band or rod-like shape. Less mature neutrophils - those that have recently been released from the bone marrow into the bloodstream - are known as "bands" or "stabs". Stab is a German term for rod.

- Lymphocytes - Higher with some viral infections such as glandular fever and. Also raised in chronic lymphocytic leukemia (CLL). Can be decreased by HIV infection. In adults, lymphocytes are the second most common WBC type after neutrophils. In young children under age 8, lymphocytes are more common than neutrophils.
- Monocytes - May be raised in bacterial infection, tuberculosis, malaria, Rocky Mountain spotted fever, monocytic leukemia, chronic ulcerative colitis and regional enteritis
- Eosinophil granulocytes - Increased in parasitic infections, asthma, or allergic reaction.
- Basophil granulocytes- May be increased in bone marrow related conditions such as leukemia or lymphoma.

A manual count will also give information about other cells that are not normally present in peripheral blood, but may be released in certain disease processes.

Platelets

- Platelet numbers are given, as well as information about their size and the range of sizes in the blood.
- Mean platelet volume (MPV) - a measurement of the average size of platelets.

Interpretation

Certain disease states are defined by an absolute increase or decrease in the number of a particular type of cell in the bloodstream. For example:

Type of Cell	Increase	Decrease
Red Blood Cells (RBC)	erythrocytosis or polycythemia	anemia or erythroblastopenia
White Blood Cells (WBC):	leukocytosis	leukopenia
-- lymphocytes	-- lymphocytosis	-- lymphocytopenia
-- granulocytes:	-- granulocytosis	-- granulocytopenia or agranulocytosis
-- --neutrophils	-- --neutrophilia	-- --neutropenia
-- --eosinophils	-- --eosinophilia	-- --eosinopenia
-- --basophils	-- --basophilia	-- --basopenia
Platelets	thrombocytosis	thrombocytopenia
All cell lines	-	pancytopenia

Many disease states are heralded by changes in the blood count:

- leukocytosis can be a sign of infection.
- thrombocytopenia can result from drug toxicity.

- pancytopenia is generally as the result of decreased production from the bone marrow, and is a common complication of cancer chemotherapy.

References

- http://www.missouricancer.com/index.jsp?page=cbc Wikipedia:Link rot
- http://www.labtestsonline.org/understanding/analytes/cbc/test.html
- http://www.bloodcountcbc.info/

Diagnosis

Schilling test

The **Schilling test** is a medical investigation used for patients with vitamin B_{12} deficiency. The purpose of the test is to determine if the patient has pernicious anemia.

It is named for Robert F. Schilling.

Process

The Schilling test has multiple stages.. As noted below, it can be done at any time after vitamin B_{12} supplementation and body store replacement, and some clinicians recommend that in severe deficiency cases, at least several weeks of vitamin repletion be done before the test (more than one B_{12} shot, and also oral folic acid), in order to insure that impaired

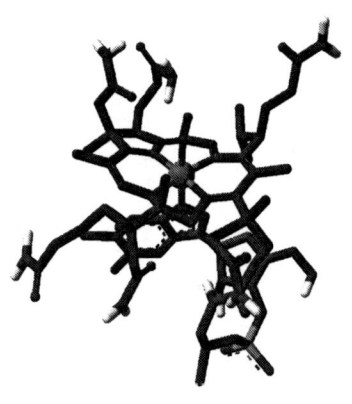

Vitamin B_{12}

absorption of B_{12} (with or without intrinsic factor) is not occurring, due to damage to the intestinal mucosa from the conditions of malabsorption arrising from B_{12} and folate deficiency themselves.

Stage 1: oral vitamin B_{12} plus intramuscular vitamin B_{12}

In the first part of the test, the patient is given radiolabeled vitamin B_{12} to drink or eat. The most commonly used radiolabels are ^{57}Co and ^{58}Co. An intramuscular injection of unlabeled vitamin B_{12} is given at or around the same time. This is not enough to replete or saturate body stores of B_{12} (this requires about 10 B_{12} injections over some length of time). The purpose of the single injection is to temporarily saturate B_{12} receptors in the liver with enough normal vitamin B_{12} to prevent radioactive vitamin B_{12} binding in body tissues (especially in the liver), so that if absorbed from the G.I. tract, it will pass into the urine. The patient's urine is then collected over the next 24 hours to assess the absorption.

Normally, the ingested radiolabeled vitamin B_{12} will be absorbed into the body. Since the body already has liver receptors for transcobalamin/vitamin B_{12} saturated by the injection, much of the ingested vitamin B_{12} will be excreted in the urine.

- A normal result shows **at least 5%** of the radiolabeled vitamin B_{12} in the urine over the first 24 hours.

- In patients with pernicious anemia or with deficiency due to impaired absorption, **less than 5%** of the radiolabeled vitamin B_{12} is detected.

Stage 2: vitamin B_{12} and intrinsic factor

If an abnormality is found, the test is repeated, this time with additional oral intrinsic factor.

- If this second urine collection is normal, this shows a lack of intrinsic factor production, or pernicious anemia.
- A low result on the second test implies abnormal intestinal absorption (malabsorption), which could be caused by coeliac disease, biliary disease, Whipple's disease, fish tapeworm infestation (Diphyllobothrium latum), or liver disease. Malabsorption of B_{12} can be caused by intestinal dysfunction from a low vitamin level in-and-of-itself (see below), causing test result confusion if repletion has not been done for some days previously.

Stage 3: vitamin B_{12} and antibiotics

This stage is useful for identifying patients with bacterial overgrowth syndrome.

Stage 4: vitamin B_{12} and pancreatic enzymes

This stage, in which pancreatic enzymes are administered, can be useful in identifying patients with pancreatitis.

Combined stage 1 and stage 2

In some versions of the Schilling's test, B_{12} can be given both with and without intrinsic factor at the same time, using different cobalt radioisotopes ^{57}Co and ^{58}Co, which have different radiation signatures, in order to differentiate the two forms of B_{12}. This allows for only a single radioactive urine collection.

Complications

Note that the B_{12} shot which begins the Schilling's test is enough to go a considerable way toward treating B_{12} deficiency, so the test is also a partial *treatment* for B_{12} deficiency. Also, the classic Schilling test can be performed at any time, even after full B_{12} repletion and correction of the anemia, and it will still show if the cause of the B_{12} deficiency was intrinsic-factor related. In fact, some clinicians have suggested that folate and B_{12} replacement for several weeks be normally performed *before* a Schilling's test is done, since folate and B_{12} deficiencies are both known to interfere with intestinal cell function, and thus cause malabsorption of B_{12} on their own, even if intrinsic factor is being made. This state would then tend to cause a false-positive test for both simple B_{12} and intrinsic factor-related B_{12} malabsorption. Several weeks of vitamin replacement are necessary, before epitheial damage to the G.I. tract from B_{12} deficiency is corrected.

Many labs have stopped performing the Schilling's test, due to lack of production of the cobalt radioisotopes and labeled-B_{12} test substances. Also, injection replacement of B_{12} has become relatively inexpensive, and can be self-administered by patients, as well as megadose oral B_{12}. Since these are the same treatments which would be administered for most causes of B_{12} malabsorption even if the exact cause were identified, the diagnostic test may be omitted without damage to the patient (so long as follow-up treatment and occasional serum B_{12} testing is not allowed to lapse).

It is possible for use of other radiopharmaceuticals to interfere with interpretation of the test.

Diagnoses

Part 1 test result	Part 2 test result	Diagnosis
Normal	-	Normal or vitamin B_{12} deficiency
Low	Normal	Pernicious anemia
Low	Low	Malabsorption

External links

• MedlinePlus Encyclopedia *003572* [1]

Diphyllobothrium

Diphyllobothrium
Proglottids of *D. latum*
Scientific classification

Kingdom:	Animalia
Phylum:	Platyhelminthes
Class:	Cestoda
Subclass:	Eucestoda
Order:	Pseudophyllidea
Family:	Diphyllobothriidae
Genus:	*Diphyllobothrium*

Species
D. latum *D. pacificum* *D. cordatum* *D. ursi* *D. dendriticum* *D. lanceolatum* *D. dalliae* *D. yonagoensis* *D. nihonkaiense=D. klebanovskii*

Diphyllobothrium is a genus of tapeworm which can cause Diphyllobothriasis in humans through consumption of raw or undercooked fish. The principal species causing diphyllobothriosis is *Diphyllobothrium latum*, known as the **broad** or **fish tapeworm**, or **broad fish tapeworm**. *D. latum* is a pseudophyllid cestode that infects fish and mammals. *D. latum* is native to Scandinavia, western Russia, and the Baltics, though it is now also present in North America, especially the Pacific Northwest. In Far East Russia, *D. klebanovskii*, having Pacific salmon as its second intermediate host, was identified. Other members of the genus *Diphyllobothrium* include *Diphyllobothrium dendriticum* (the salmon tapeworm), which has a much larger range (the whole northern hemisphere), *D. pacificum*, *D. cordatum*, *D. ursi*, *D. lanceolatum*, *D. dalliae*, and *D. yonagoensis*, all of which infect humans only infrequently. In Japan, the most common species in human infection is *D. nihonkaiense*, which was only identified as a separate species from *D. latum* in 1986. It was indicated to be synonymous to *D. klebanovskii* from the molecular study.

History

The fish tapeworm has a long documented history of infecting people who regularly consume fish and especially those whose customs include the consumption of raw or undercooked fish. In the 1970s, most of the known cases of diphyllobothriasis came from Europe (5 million cases), and Asia (4 million cases) with fewer cases coming from North America and South America, and no reliable data on cases from Africa or Australia . Interestingly, despite the relatively small number of cases seen today in South America, some of the earliest archeological evidence of diphyllobothriasis comes from sites in South America. Evidence of *Diphyllobothrium spp.* has been found in 4,000-10,000 year old human remains on the western coast of South America . There is no clear point in time when *Diphyllobothrium latum* and related species were "discovered" in humans, but it is clear that diphyllobothriasis has been endemic in human populations for a very long time. Due to the changing dietary habits in many parts of the world, autochthonous, or locally-acquired, cases of diphyllobothriasis have recently been documented in previously non-endemic areas, such as Brazil . In this way, diphyllobothriasis represents an emerging infectious disease in certain parts of the world where cultural practices involving eating raw or undercooked fish are being introduced.

Morphology

The adult worm is composed of three fairly distinct morphological segments: the scolex (head), the neck, and the lower body. Each side of the scolex has a slit-like groove, which is a bothrium (tentacle) for attachment to the intestine. The scolex attaches to the neck, or proliferative region. From the neck, grows many proglottid segments which contain the reproductive organs of the worm. *D. latum* is the longest tapeworm in humans, averaging ten meters long. Adults can shed up to a million eggs a day.

In adults, proglottids are wider than they are long (hence the name *broad tapeworm*). As in all pseudophyllid cestodes, the genital pores open midventrally.

Life cycle

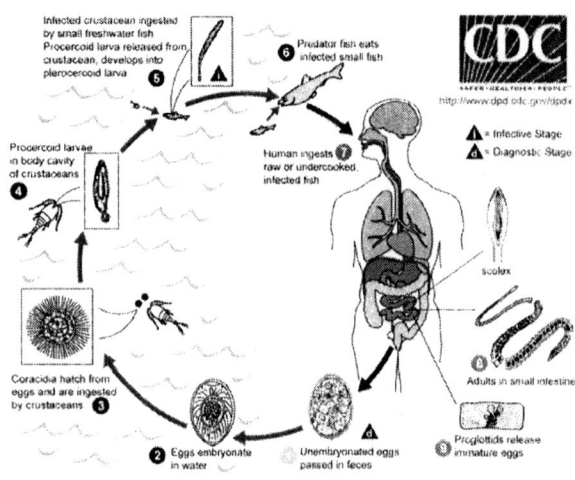

Life cycle of *D. latum*. Click the image to see full-size.

Adult tapeworms may infect humans, canids, felines, bears, pinnipeds, and mustelids, though the accuracy of the records for some of the nonhuman species is disputed. Immature eggs are passed in feces of the mammal host (the definitive host, where the worms reproduce). After ingestion by a suitable freshwater crustacean such as a copepod (the first intermediate host), the coracidia develop into procercoid larvae. Following ingestion of the copepod by a suitable second intermediate host, typically a minnow or other small freshwater fish, the procercoid larvae are released from the crustacean and migrate into the fish's flesh where they develop into a plerocercoid larvae (sparganum). The plerocercoid larvae are the infective stage for the definitive host (including humans).

Because humans do not generally eat undercooked minnows and similar small freshwater fish, these do not represent an important source of infection. Nevertheless, these small second intermediate hosts can be eaten by larger predator species, for example, trout, perch, and walleyed pike. In this case, the sparganum can migrate to the musculature of the larger predator fish and mammals can acquire the disease by eating these later intermediate infected host fish raw or undercooked. After ingestion of the infected fish, the plerocercoids develop into immature adults and then into mature adult tapeworms which will reside in the small intestine. The adults attach to the intestinal mucosa by means of the two bilateral grooves (bothria) of their scolex. The adults can reach more than 10 m (up to 30 ft) in length in some species such as *D. latum,* with more than 3,000 proglottids. One or several of the tape-like proglottid segments (hence the name tape-worm) regularly detach from the main body of the worm and release immature eggs in fresh water to start the cycle over again. Immature eggs are discharged from the proglottids (up to 1,000,000 eggs per day per worm) and are passed in the feces. The incubation period in humans, after which eggs begin to appear in the feces is typically 4–6 weeks, but can vary from as short as 2 weeks to as long as 2 years. The tapeworm can live up to 20 years.

Clinical symptoms, including occasional parasite-induced B$_{12}$ deficiency

Symptoms of diphyllobothriasis are generally mild, and can include diarrhea, abdominal pain, vomiting, weight loss, fatigue, constipation and discomfort. Approximately four out of five cases are asymptomatic and may go many years without being detected. In a small number of cases, this leads to severe vitamin B$_{12}$ deficiency due to the parasite absorbing 80% or more of the host's B$_{12}$ intake, and a megaloblastic anemia indistinguishable from pernicious anemia. The anemia can also lead to subtle demyelinative neurological symptoms (subacute combined degeneration of spinal cord). Infection for many years is ordinarily required to deplete the human body of vitamin B-12 to the point that neurological symptoms appear.

Diagnosis

Diagnosis is usually made by identifying proglottid segments, or characteristic eggs in the feces. These simple diagnostic techniques are able to identify the nature of the infection to the genus level, which is usually sufficient in a clinical setting. However, when the species needs to be determined (in epidemiological studies, for example), restriction fragment length polymorphisms can be effectively used. PCR can be performed on samples of purified eggs, or native fecal samples following sonication of the eggs to release their contents.

Treatment

Upon diagnosis, treatment is quite simple and effective. The standard treatment for diphyllobothriasis, as well as many other tapeworm infections is a single dose of Praziquantel, 5–10 mg/kg PO once for both adults and children. An alternative treatment is Niclosamide, 2 g PO once for adults or 50 mg/kg PO once . Another interesting potential diagnostic tool and treatment is the contrast medium, Gastrografin, introduced into the duodenum, which allows both visualization of the parasite, and has also been shown to cause detachment and passing of the whole worm .

Side effects of treatment

Praziquantel has few side effects, many of which are similar to the symptoms of diphyllobothriasis. They include malaise, headache, dizziness, abdominal discomfort, nausea, rise in temperature and occasionally allergic skin reactions. The side effects of Niclosamide are very rare, due to the fact that it is not absorbed in the gastrointestinal tract.

Epidemiology

People at high risk for infection have traditionally been those who regularly consume raw fish, including fishermen who eat the raw liver or roe of their catches and women preparing and tasting foods that contain raw fish. Many regional cuisines include raw or undercooked food, including sushi and sashimi in Japanese cuisine, carpaccio di persico in Italian, tartare maison in French-speaking populations, ceviche in Latin American cuisine and marinated herring in Scandinavia. With emigration and globalization, the practice of eating raw fish in these and other dishes has brought diphyllobothriasis to new parts of the world and created new endemic foci of disease.

Public health strategies

The most viable interventions include: prevention of water contamination both by raising public awareness of the dangers of defecating in recreational bodies of water and by implementation of basic sanitation measures; screening and successful treatment of people infected with the parasite; and prevention of infection of humans via consumption of raw, infected fish. The last of these can most easily be changed via education about proper preparation of fish. Fish that is thoroughly cooked, brined, or frozen at -10°C for 24–48 hours can be consumed without risk of D. latum infection.

See also

- List of parasites (human)

References

- "DPDx - Diphyllobothriasis" [1]. *CDC Division of Parasitic Diseases.*
- "UDiphyllobothrium spp." [2]. *Bad Bug Book.* Retrieved 2009-07-13.
- Janovy, John; Roberts, Larry S. (2005). *Foundations of Parasitology* (7th ed.). McGraw-Hill Education (ISE Editions). ISBN 0-07-111271-5.

External links

- http://www.stanford.edu/class/humbio103/parasites.htm

Treatment

Vitamin B

Vitamin B12

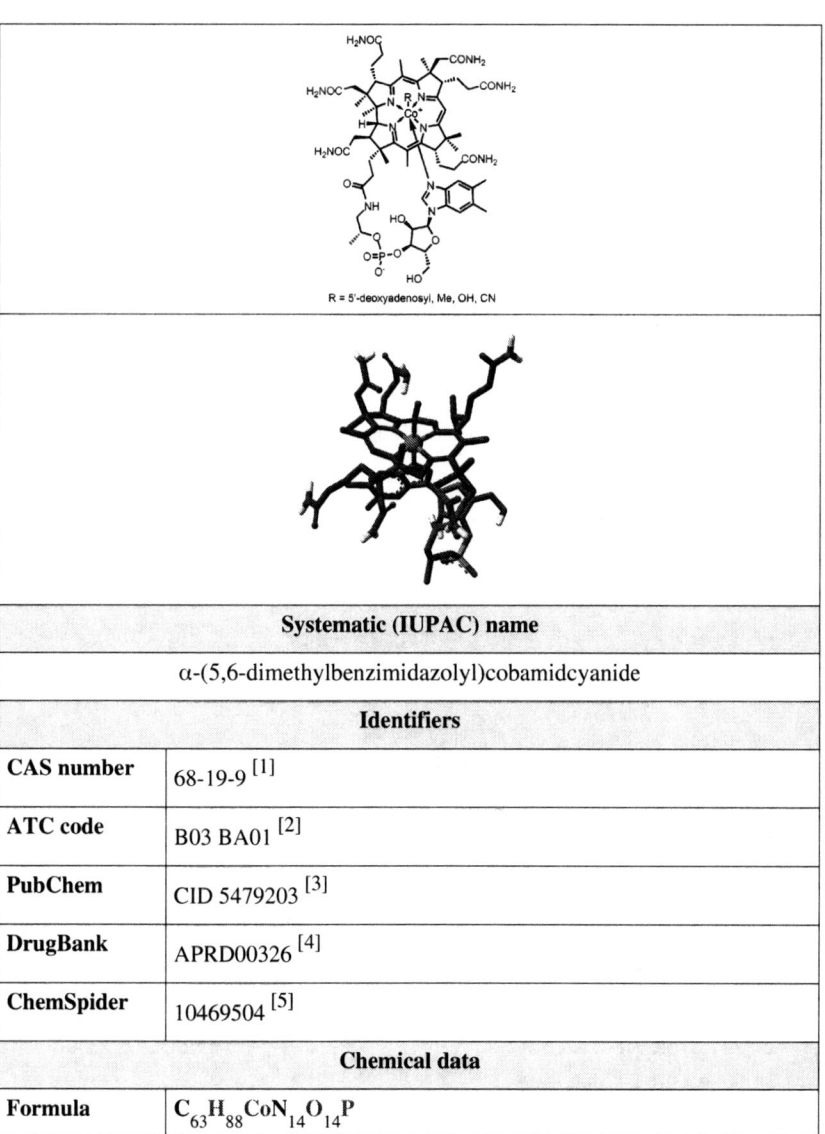

R = 5'-deoxyadenosyl, Me, OH, CN

Systematic (IUPAC) name	
α-(5,6-dimethylbenzimidazolyl)cobamidcyanide	
Identifiers	
CAS number	68-19-9 [1]
ATC code	B03 BA01 [2]
PubChem	CID 5479203 [3]
DrugBank	APRD00326 [4]
ChemSpider	10469504 [5]
Chemical data	
Formula	$C_{63}H_{88}CoN_{14}O_{14}P$

Mol. mass	1355.37 g/mol
Pharmacokinetic data	
Bioavailability	readily absorbed in distal half of the ileum
Protein binding	Very high to specific transcobalamins plasma proteins Binding of hydroxocobalamin is slightly higher than cyanocobalamin.
Metabolism	hepatic
Half-life	Approximately 6 days (400 days in the liver)
Excretion	renal
Therapeutic considerations	
Pregnancy cat.	?
Legal status	POM (UK)
Routes	oral, iv

Vitamin B$_{12}$, **vitamin B12** or **vitamin B-12**, also called **cobalamin**, is a water soluble vitamin with a key role in the normal functioning of the brain and nervous system, and for the formation of blood. It is one of the eight B vitamins. It is normally involved in the metabolism of every cell of the human body, especially affecting DNA synthesis and regulation, but also fatty acid synthesis and energy production. As the largest and most structurally complicated vitamin, it can be produced industrially only through bacterial fermentation-synthesis.

Vitamin B$_{12}$ consists of a class of chemically-related compounds (vitamers), all of which have vitamin activity. It contains the biochemically rare element cobalt. Biosynthesis of the basic structure of the vitamin in nature is only accomplished by simple organisms such as some bacteria and algae, but conversion between different forms of the vitamin can be accomplished in the human body. A common synthetic form of the vitamin, cyanocobalamin, does not occur in nature, but is used in many pharmaceuticals and supplements, and as a food additive, because of its stability and lower cost. In the body it is converted to the physiological forms, methylcobalamin and adenosylcobalamin, leaving behind the cyanide, albeit in minimal concentration. More recently, hydroxocobalamin (a form produced by bacteria), methylcobalamin, and adenosylcobalamin can also be found in more expensive pharmacological products and food supplements. The utility of these is presently debated.

Vitamin B$_{12}$ was discovered from its relationship to the disease pernicious anemia, which is an autoimmune disease that destroys parietal cells in the stomach that secrete intrinsic factor. Intrinsic factor is crucial for the normal absorption of B$_{12}$, so a lack of intrinsic factor, as seen in pernicious anemia, causes a vitamin B$_{12}$ deficiency. Many other subtler kinds of vitamin B$_{12}$ deficiency and their biochemical effects have since been elucidated.

Terminology

The names **vitamin B$_{12}$** or **vitamin B12** or **vitamin B-12**, which are sometimes shortened to **B$_{12}$** or **B12**, and the alternative name cyanocobalamin generally refer to all forms of the vitamin. Some medical practitioners have suggested that its use be split into two different categories, however.

- In a broad sense, B$_{12}$ refers to a group of cobalt-containing vitamer compounds known as cobalamins: these include cyanocobalamin (an artifact formed as a result of the use of cyanide in the purification procedures), hydroxocobalamin (another medicinal form, produced by bacteria), and finally, the two naturally occurring cofactor forms of B$_{12}$ in the human body: 5'-deoxyadenosylcobalamin (adenosylcobalamin—AdoB12), the cofactor of Methylmalonyl Coenzyme A mutase (MUT), and methylcobalamin (MeB$_{12}$), the cofactor of 5-methyltetrahydrofolate-homocysteine methyltransferase (MTR).

- The term B$_{12}$ may be properly used to refer to cyanocobalamin, the principal B$_{12}$ form used for foods and in nutritional supplements. This ordinarily creates no problem, except perhaps in rare cases of eye nerve damage, where the body is only marginally able to use this form due to high cyanide levels in the blood due to cigarette smoking, and thus requires cessation of smoking, or else B$_{12}$ given in another form, for the optic symptoms to abate. However, tobacco amblyopia is a rare enough condition that debate continues about whether or not it represents a peculiar B$_{12}$ deficiency which is resistant to treatment with cyanocobalamin.

Finally, so-called **pseudo-B$_{12}$** refers to B$_{12}$-like substances which are found in certain organisms, including *Spirulina* (a cyanobacterium) and some algae. These substances are active in tests of B$_{12}$ activity by highly sensitive antibody-binding serum assay tests, which measure levels of B$_{12}$ and B$_{12}$-like compounds in blood. However, these substances do not have B$_{12}$ biological activity for humans, a fact which may pose a danger to vegans and others on limited diets who do not ingest B$_{12}$ producing bacteria, but who nevertheless may show normal "B$_{12}$" levels in the standard immunoassay which has become the normal medical method for testing for B$_{12}$ deficiency.

Structure

Vitamin B$_{12}$ is a collection of cobalt and corrin ring molecules which are defined by their particular vitamin function in the body. All of the substrate cobalt-corrin molecules from which B$_{12}$ is made must be synthesized by bacteria. However, after this synthesis is complete, the body has a limited power to convert any form of B$_{12}$ to another, by means of enzymatically removing certain prosthetic chemical groups from the cobalt atom. The various forms (vitamers) of B$_{12}$ are all deeply red colored, due to the color of the cobalt-corrin complex.

Cyanocobalamin is one such "vitamer" in this B complex, because it can be metabolized in the body to an active co-enzyme form. However, the cyanocobalamin form of B$_{12}$ does not occur in nature normally, but is a byproduct of the fact that other forms of B$_{12}$ are avid binders of cyanide (-CN) which they pick up in the process of activated charcoal purification of the vitamin after it is made by bacteria in the commercial process. Since the cyanocobalamin form of B_{12} is easy to crystallize and is not sensitive to air-oxidation, it is typically used as a form of B_{12} for food additives and in many common multivitamins. However, this form is not perfectly synonymous with B_{12}, in as much as a number of substances (vitamers) have B_{12} vitamin activity and can properly be labeled vitamin B_{12}, and cyanocobalamin is but one of them. (Thus, all cyanocobalamin is vitamin B_{12}, but not all vitamin B_{12} is cyanocobalamin).

Hydroxocobalamin is another form of B_{12} commonly encountered in pharmacology, but which is not normally present in the human body. Hydroxocobalamin is sometimes denonoted B_{12a}. This form of B_{12} is the form produced by bacteria, and is what is converted to cyanocobalmin in the commercial charcoal filtration step of production. Hydroxocobalamin has an avid affinity for cyanide ion and has been used as an antidote to cyanide poisoning. It is supplied typically in water solution for injection. Hydroxocobalamin is thought to be converted to the active enzymic forms of B_{12} more easily than cyanocobalamin, and since it is little more expensive than cyanocobalamin, and has longer retention times in the body, has been used for vitamin replacement in situations where added reassurance of activity is desired. Intramuscular administration of hydroxocobalamin is also the preferred treatment for pediatric patients with intrinsic cobalamin metabolic diseases, for vitamin B_{12} deficient patients with tobacco amblyopia (which is thought to perhaps have a component of cyanide poisoning from cyanide in cigarette smoke); and for treatment of patients with pernicious anemia who have optic neuropathy.

B_{12} is the most chemically complex of all the vitamins. The structure of B_{12} is based on a corrin ring, which is similar to the porphyrin ring found in heme, chlorophyll, and cytochrome. The central metal ion is cobalt. Four of the six coordination sites are provided by the corrin ring, and a fifth by a dimethylbenzimidazole group. The sixth coordination site, the center of reactivity, is variable, being a cyano group (-CN), a hydroxyl group (-OH), a methyl group (-CH$_3$) or a 5'-deoxyadenosyl group (here the C5' atom of the deoxyribose forms the covalent bond with Co), respectively, to yield the four B_{12} forms mentioned above. Historically, the covalent C-Co bond is one of first examples of carbon-metal bonds to be discovered in biology. The hydrogenases and, by necessity, enzymes associated with cobalt utilization, involve metal-carbon bonds.

Synthesis

Neither plants nor animals are independently capable of constructing vitamin B_{12}. Only bacteria have the enzymes required for its synthesis. The total synthesis of B_{12} was reported by Robert Burns Woodward and Albert Eschenmoser in 1972, and remains one of the classic feats of organic synthesis. Species from the following genera are known to synthesize B_{12}: *Aerobacter, Agrobacterium, Alcaligenes, Azotobacter, Bacillus, Clostridium, Corynebacterium, Flavobacterium, Micromonospora, Mycobacterium, Nocardia, Propionibacterium, Protaminobacter, Proteus, Pseudomonas, Rhizobium,*

Salmonella, *Serratia*, *Streptomyces*, *Streptococcus* and *Xanthomonas*.

Industrial production of B_{12} is through fermentation of selected microorganisms. *Streptomyces griseus*, a bacterium once thought to be a yeast, was the commercial source of vitamin B_{12} for many years. The species *Pseudomonas denitrificans* and *Propionibacterium shermanii* are more commonly used today. These are frequently grown under special conditions to enhance yield, and at least one company, Rhône-Poulenc of France, at one point used genetically engineered versions of one or both of these species. It is not clear whether Sanofi-Aventis, the company into which the pharmaceutical division of Rhône-Poulenc merged, has continued the use of genetically modified organisms.

Functions

Vitamin B_{12} is normally involved in the metabolism of every cell of the body, especially affecting the DNA synthesis and regulation but also fatty acid synthesis and energy production. However, many (though not all) of the effects of functions of B_{12} can be replaced by sufficient quantities of folic acid (vitamin B_9), since B_{12} is used to regenerate folate in the body. Most vitamin B_{12} deficiency symptoms are actually folate deficiency symptoms, since they

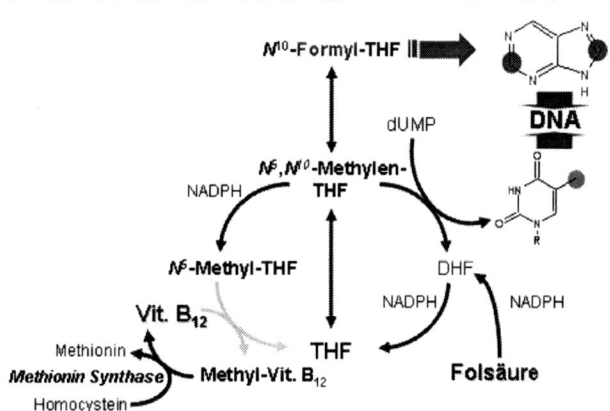

Metabolism of folic acid. The role of Vitamin B_{12} is seen at bottom-left.

include all the effects of pernicious anemia and megaloblastosis, which are due to poor synthesis of DNA when the body does not have a proper supply of folic acid for the production of thymine. When sufficient folic acid is available, all known B_{12} related deficiency syndromes normalize, save those narrowly connected with the vitamin B_{12}-dependent enzymes MUT, and 5-methyltetrahydrofolate-homocysteine methyltransferase (MTR), also known as methionine synthase; and the buildup of their respective substrates (methylmalonic acid, MMA) and homocysteine.

Coenzyme B_{12}'s reactive C-Co bond participates in three main types of enzyme-catalyzed reactions.

1. **Isomerases**. Rearrangements in which a hydrogen atom is directly transferred between two adjacent atoms with concomitant exchange of the second substituent, X, which may be a carbon atom with substituents, an oxygen atom of an alcohol, or an amine.
2. **Methyltransferases**. Methyl (-CH$_3$) group transfers between two molecules.
3. **Dehalogenases**. Reactions in which a halogen atom is removed from an organic molecule. Enzymes in this class have not been identified in humans.

In humans, two major coenzyme B$_{12}$-dependent enzyme families corresponding to the first two reaction types, are known. These are typified by the following two enzymes:

1. MUT is an isomerase which uses the AdoB$_{12}$ form and reaction type 1 to catalyze a carbon skeleton rearrangement (the X group is -COSCoA). MUT's reaction converts MMl-CoA to Su-CoA, an important step in the extraction of energy from proteins and fats *(for more see MUT's reaction mechanism)*. This functionality is lost in vitamin B$_{12}$ deficiency, and can be measured clinically as an increased methylmalonic acid (MMA) level. Unfortunately, an elevated MMA, though sensitive to B$_{12}$ deficiency, is probably overly sensitive, and not all who have it actually have B$_{12}$ deficiency. For example, MMA is elevated in 90–98% of patients with B$_{12}$ deficiency; however 20–25% of patients over the age of 70 have elevated levels of MMA, yet 25–33% of them do not have B$_{12}$ deficiency. For this reason, assessment of MMA levels is not routinely recommended in the elderly. There is no "gold standard" test for B$_{12}$ deficiency because as a B$_{12}$ deficiency occurs, serum values may be maintained while tissue B$_{12}$ stores become depleted. Therefore, serum B$_{12}$ values above the cut-off point of deficiency do not necessarily indicate adequate B$_{12}$ status The MUT function cannot be affected by folate supplementation, which is necessary for myelin synthesis (see mechanism below) and certain other functions of the central nervous system. Other functions of B$_{12}$ related to DNA synthesis related to MTR dysfunction (see below) can often be corrected with supplementation with the vitamin folic acid, but not the elevated levels of homocysteine, which is normally converted to methionine by MTR.

2. MTR, also known as methionine synthase, is a methyltransferase enzyme, which uses the MeB$_{12}$ and reaction type 2 to catalyze the conversion of the amino acid homocysteine (Hcy) back into methionine (Met) *(for more see MTR's reaction mechanism)*. This functionality is lost in vitamin B$_{12}$ deficiency, and can be measured clinically as an increased homocysteine level *in vitro*. Increased homocysteine can also be caused by a folic acid deficiency, since B$_{12}$ helps to regenerate the tetrahydrofolate (THF) active form of folic acid. Without B$_{12}$, folate is trapped as 5-methyl-folate, from which THF cannot be recovered unless a MTR process reacts the 5-methyl-folate with homocysteine to produce methionine and THF, thus decreasing the need for fresh sources of THF from the diet. THF may be produced in the conversion of homocysteine to methionine, or may be obtained in the diet. It is converted by a non-B$_{12}$-dependent process to 5,10-methylene-THF, which is involved in the synthesis of thymine. Reduced availability of 5,10-methylene-THF results in problems with DNA synthesis, and ultimately in ineffective production cells with rapid turnover, in particular blood cells, and also intestinal wall cells which are responsible for absorption. The failure of blood cell production results in the once-dreaded and fatal disease, pernicious anemia. All of the DNA synthetic effects, including the megaloblastic anemia of pernicious anemia, resolve if sufficient folate is present (since levels of 5,10-methylene-THF still remain adequate with enough dietary folate). Thus the best-known "function" of B$_{12}$ (that which is involved with DNA synthesis, cell-division, and anemia) is actually a facultative function which is mediated by B$_{12}$-conservation of an active form of folate which is needed for efficient DNA

production. Other cobalamin-requiring methyltransferase enzymes are also known in bacteria, such as Me-H4-MPT, coenzyme M methyl transferase.

Specific MUT and MTR failure syndromes, even with excess folate

If folate is present in quantity, then of the two absolutely vitamin B$_{12}$-dependent enzyme-family reactions in humans, the MUT-family reactions show the most direct and characteristic secondary effects, focusing on the nervous system (see below). This is because the MTR (methyltransferase-type) reactions are involved in regenerating folate, and thus are less evident when folate is in good supply.

Since the late 1990s, folic acid has begun to be added to fortify flour in many countries, so folate deficiency is now more rare. At the same time, since DNA synthetic-sensitive tests for anemia and erythrocyte size are routinely done in even simple medical test clinics (so that these folate-mediated biochemical effects are more often directly detected), the MTR-dependent effects of B$_{12}$ deficiency are becoming apparent not as anemia due to DNA-synthetic problems (as they were classically), but now mainly as a simple and less obvious elevation of homocysteine in the blood and urine (homocysteinuria). This condition may result in long term damage to arteries and in clotting (stroke and heart attack), but this effect is difficult to separate from other common processes associated with atherosclerosis and aging.

The specific myelin damage resulting from B$_{12}$ deficiency, even in the presence of adequate folate and methionine, is more specifically and clearly a vitamin deficiency problem. It has been connected to B$_{12}$ most directly by reactions related to MUT, which is absolutely required to convert methylmalonyl coenzyme A into succinyl coenzyme A. Failure of this second reaction to occur results in elevated levels of MMA, a myelin destabilizer. Excessive MMA will prevent normal fatty acid synthesis, or it will be incorporated into fatty acid itself rather than normal malonic acid. If this abnormal fatty acid subsequently is incorporated into myelin, the resulting myelin will be too fragile, and demyelination will occur. Although the precise mechanism(s) are not known with certainty, the result is subacute combined degeneration of central nervous system and spinal cord. Whatever the cause, it is known that B$_{12}$ deficiency causes neuropathies, even if folic acid is present in good supply, and therefore anemia is not present.

Vitamin B$_{12}$-dependent MTR reactions may also have neurological effects, through an indirect mechanism. Adequate methionine (which, like folate, must otherwise be obtained in the diet, if it is not regenerated from homocysteine by a B$_{12}$ dependent reaction) is needed to make S-adenosyl-methionine (SAMe), which is in turn necessary for methylation of myelin sheath phospholipids. Although production of SAMe is not B$_{12}$ dependent, help in recycling for provision of one adequate substrate for it (the essential amino acid methionine) is assisted by B$_{12}$. In addition, SAMe is involved in the manufacture of certain neurotransmitters, catecholamines and in brain metabolism. These neurotransmitters are important for maintaining mood, possibly explaining why depression is associated with B$_{12}$ deficiency. Methylation of the myelin sheath phospholipids may also depend on adequate folate, which in turn is dependent on MTR recycling, unless ingested in relatively high amounts.

Human absorption and distribution

The human physiology of vitamin B_{12} is complex, and therefore is prone to mishaps leading to vitamin B_{12} deficiency. Unlike most nutrients, absorption of vitamin B_{12} actually begins in the mouth, where small amounts of unbound crystalline B_{12} can be absorbed through the mucous membrane. Food protein-bound vitamin B_{12} is digested in the stomach by proteolytic gastric enzymes, which require an acid pH. In addition, antacid drugs may also inhibit the efficacy of gastric acids in this process.

B_{12} taken in a low-solubility, non-chewable supplement pill form may bypass the mouth and stomach and not mix with gastric acids, but these are not necessary for the absorption of free B_{12} not bound to protein.

Recently available sublingual methylcobalamin has been available in 1 mg tablets. Such tablets have higher bioavailability than the older cyanocobalamin. No cyanide is released with methylcobolamin making it safer. http://www.efsa.europa.eu/EFSA/efsa_locale-1178620753812_1211902125049.htm

Once the B_{12} is freed from the proteins in food, R-proteins, such as haptocorrins and cobalaphilins, are secreted, which bind to free vitamin B_{12} to form a B_{12}-R complex. Also in the stomach, intrinsic factor (IF), a protein synthesized by gastric parietal cells, is secreted in response to histamine, gastrin and pentagastrin, as well as the presence of food. If this step fails due to gastric parietal cell atrophy (the problem in pernicious anemia), sufficient B_{12} is not absorbed later on, unless administered orally in relatively massive doses (0.5 to 1 mg/day). Due to the complexity of B_{12} absorption, geriatric patients, many of whom are hypoacidic due to reduced parietal cell function, have an increased risk of B_{12} deficiency.

In the duodenum, proteases digest R-proteins and release B_{12}, which then binds to IF, to form a complex (IF/B_{12}). B_{12} must be attached to IF for it to be absorbed, as receptors on the enterocytes in the terminal ileum of the small bowel only recognize the B_{12}-IF complex; in addition, intrinsic factor protects the vitamin from catabolism by intestinal bacteria. Therefore, absorption of food vitamin B_{12} requires an intact and functioning stomach, exocrine pancreas, intrinsic factor, and small bowel. Problems with any one of these organs makes a vitamin B_{12} deficiency possible. Individuals who lack intrinsic factor have a decreased ability to absorb B_{12}. This results in 80–100% excretion of oral doses in the feces versus 30–60% excretion in feces as seen in individuals with adequate IF.

Once the IF/B_{12} complex is recognized by specialized ileal receptors, it is transported into the portal circulation. The vitamin is then transferred to transcobalamin II (TC-II/B_{12}), which serves as the plasma transporter. Hereditary defects in production of the transcobalamins and their receptors may produce functional deficiencies in B_{12} and infantile megaloblastic anemia, and abnormal B_{12} related biochemistry, even in some cases with normal blood B$_{12}$ levels. For the vitamin to serve inside cells, the TC-II/B$_{12}$ complex must bind to a cell receptor, and be endocytosed. The transcobalamin-II is degraded within a lysosome, and free B$_{12}$ is finally released into the cytoplasm, where it may be transformed into the proper coenzyme, by certain cellular enzymes (see above).

The total amount of vitamin B$_{12}$ stored in body is about 2–5 mg in adults. Around 50% of this is stored in the liver. Approximately 0.1% of this is lost per day by secretions into the gut, as not all these secretions are reabsorbed. Bile is the main form of B$_{12}$ excretion; however, most of the B$_{12}$ secreted in the bile is recycled via enterohepatic circulation. Due to the extremely efficient enterohepatic circulation of B$_{12}$, the liver can store several years' worth of vitamin B$_{12}$; therefore, nutritional deficiency of this vitamin is rare. How fast B$_{12}$ levels change depends on the balance between how much B$_{12}$ is obtained from the diet, how much is secreted and how much is absorbed. B$_{12}$ deficiency may arise in a year if initial stores are low and genetic factors unfavourable, or may not appear for decades. In infants, B$_{12}$ deficiency can appear much more quickly.

History

B$_{12}$ deficiency is the cause of pernicious anemia, an anemic disease that was usually fatal and had unknown etiology when it was first described in medicine. The cure, and B$_{12}$, were discovered by accident. George Whipple had been doing experiments in which he induced anemia in dogs by bleeding them, and then fed them various foods to observe which diets allowed them fastest recovery from the anemia produced. In the process, he discovered that ingesting large amounts of liver seemed to most-rapidly cure the anemia of blood loss. Thus, he hypothesized that liver ingestion might treat pernicious anemia. He tried this and reported some signs of success in 1920.

After a series of careful clinical studies, George Richards Minot and William Murphy set out to partly isolate the substance in liver which cured anemia in dogs, and found that it was iron. They also found that an entirely different liver substance cured pernicious anemia in humans, that had no effect on dogs under the conditions used. The specific factor treatment for pernicious anemia, found in liver juice, had been found by this coincidence. Minot and Murphy reported these experiments in 1926. This was the first real progress with this disease. Despite this discovery, for several years patients were still required to eat large amounts of raw liver or to drink considerable amounts of liver juice.

In 1928, the chemist Edwin Cohn prepared a liver extract that was 50 to 100 times more potent than the natural liver products. The extract was the first workable treatment for the disease. For their initial work in pointing the way to a working treatment, Whipple, Minot, and Murphy shared the 1934 Nobel Prize in Physiology or Medicine.

These events in turn eventually led to discovery of the soluble vitamin, called vitamin B$_{12}$, in the liver juice. The vitamin in liver extracts was not isolated until 1948 by the chemists Karl A. Folkers of the United States and Alexander R. Todd of Great Britain. The substance proved to be cobalamin—the most complex of all the vitamins. It could also be injected directly into muscle, making it possible to treat pernicious anemia more easily.

The chemical structure of the molecule was determined by Dorothy Crowfoot Hodgkin and her team in 1956, based on crystallographic data. Eventually, methods of producing the vitamin in large quantities from bacteria cultures were developed in the 1950s, and these led to the modern form of treatment for the disease.

Symptoms and damage from deficiency

Main article: Vitamin B12 deficiency

Vitamin B_{12} deficiency can potentially cause severe and irreversible damage, especially to the brain and nervous system. At levels only slightly lower than normal, a range of symptoms such as fatigue, depression, and poor memory may be experienced. However, these symptoms by themselves are too nonspecific to diagnose deficiency of the vitamin.

Vitamin B_{12} deficiency can also cause symptoms of mania and psychosis.

Vitamin B_{12} deficiency has the following pathomorphology and symptoms:

Pathomorphology: A spongiform state of neural tissue along with edema of fibers and deficiency of tissue. The myelin decays, along with axial fiber. In later phases, fibric sclerosis of nervous tissues occurs. Those changes apply to dorsal parts of the spinal cord and to pyramidal tracts in lateral cords. The pathophysiologic state of the spinal cord is called subacute combined degeneration of spinal cord.

In the brain itself, changes are less severe: They occur as small sources of nervous fibers decay and accumulation of astrocytes, usually subcortically located, and also round hemorrhages with a torus of glial cells. Pathological changes can be noticed as well in the posterior roots of the cord and, to lesser extent, in peripheral nerves.

Clinical symptoms: The main syndrome of vitamin B_{12} deficiency is Biermer's disease (pernicious anemia). It is characterized by a triad of symptoms:

1. Anemia with bone marrow promegaloblastosis (megaloblastic anemia)
2. Gastrointestinal symptoms
3. Neurological symptoms

Each of those symptoms can occur either alone or along with others. The neurological complex, defined as *myelosis funicularis*, consists of the following symptoms:

1. Impaired perception of deep touch, pressure and vibration, abolishment of sense of touch, very annoying and persistent paresthesias
2. Ataxia of dorsal cord type
3. Decrease or abolishment of deep muscle-tendon reflexes
4. Pathological reflexes — Babinski, Rossolimo and others, also severe paresis

During the course of disease, mental disorders can occur. These include irritability, focus/concentration problems, depressive state with suicidal tendencies, and paraphrenia complex. These symptoms may not reverse after correction of hematological abnormalities, and the chance of complete reversal decreases with the length of time the neurological symptoms have been present.

Sources

Foods

Ultimately, animals must obtain vitamin B$_{12}$ directly or indirectly from bacteria, and these bacteria may inhabit a section of the gut which is posterior to the section where B$_{12}$ is absorbed. Thus, herbivorous animals must either obtain B$_{12}$ from bacteria in their rumens, or (if fermenting plant material in the hindgut) by reingestion of cecotrope fæces.

Vitamin B$_{12}$ is found in foods that come from animals, including fish and shellfish, meat (especially liver), poultry, eggs, milk, and milk products. One half chicken breast provides some 0.3 µg (micrograms) per serving or 6.0% of one's daily value (DV); 85 grams (3 oz) of beef, 2.4 µg, or 40% of one's DV; one slice of liver 47.9 µg or 780% of DV; and 85 grams (3 oz) of molluscs 84.1 µg, or 1,400% of DV.

Eggs are often mentioned as a good B$_{12}$ source, but they also contain a factor (avidin) that blocks absorption. Certain insects such as termites contain B$_{12}$ produced by their gut bacteria, in a way analogous to ruminant animals. An NIH Fact Sheet lists a variety of food sources of vitamin B$_{12}$.

While lacto-ovo vegetarians usually get enough B$_{12}$ through consuming dairy products, vegans will lack B$_{12}$ unless they consume multivitamin supplements or B$_{12}$-fortified foods. Examples of fortified foods include fortified breakfast cereals, fortified soy products, fortified energy bars, and fortified nutritional yeast. According to the UK Vegan Society, the present consensus is that any B$_{12}$ present in plant foods is likely to be unavailable to humans because B$_{12}$ analogues can compete with B$_{12}$ and inhibit metabolism.

Claimed sources of B$_{12}$ that have been shown to be inadequate or unreliable through direct studies of vegans include laver (a seaweed), barley grass, and human gut bacteria.

Supplements

Vitamin B$_{12}$ is provided as a supplement in many processed foods, and is also available in vitamin pill form, including multi-vitamins. Vitamin B$_{12}$ can be supplemented in healthy subjects also by liquid, transdermal patch, nasal spray, or injection and is available singly or in combination with other supplements.

Cyanocobalamin is converted to its active forms, first hydroxocobalamin and then methylcobalamin and adenosylcobalamin in the liver.

The sublingual route, in which B$_{12}$ is presumably or supposedly absorbed more directly under the tongue, has not proven to be necessary or helpful, though there are a number of lozenges, pills, and even a lollipop designed for sublingual absorption. A 2003 study found no significant difference in absorption for serum levels from oral vs. sublingual delivery of 0.5 mg of cobalamin. Sublingual methods of replacement are effective only because of the typically high doses (0.5 mg), which are swallowed, not because of placement of the tablet. As noted below, such very high doses of oral B$_{12}$ may be effective as treatments, even if gastro-intestinal tract absorption is impaired by gastric atrophy (pernicious anemia).

Injection and patches are sometimes used if digestive absorption is impaired, but there is evidence that this course of action may not be necessary with modern high potency oral supplements (such as 0.5 to 1 mg or more). Even pernicious anemia can be treated entirely by the oral route. These supplements carry such large doses of the vitamin that 1% to 5% of high oral doses of free crystalline B$_{12}$ is absorbed along the entire intestine by passive diffusion.

However, if the patient has inborn errors in the methyltransfer pathway (cobalamin C disease, combined methylmalonic aciduria and homocystinuria), treatment with intravenous, intramuscular hydroxocobalamin or transdermal B$_{12}$ is needed.

Cyanocobalamin is also sometimes added to beverages including Diet Coke Plus and many energy drinks.

Recommendations

The Dietary Reference Intake for an adult ranges from 2 to 3 µg per day.

Vitamin B$_{12}$ is believed to be safe when used orally in amounts that do not exceed the recommended dietary allowance (RDA). The RDA for vitamin B$_{12}$ in pregnant women is 2.6 µg per day and 2.8 µg during lactation periods. There is insufficient reliable information available about the safety of consuming greater amounts of vitamin B$_{12}$ during pregnancy.

The Vegan Society, the Vegetarian Resource Group, and the Physicians Committee for Responsible Medicine, among others, recommend that vegans either consistently eat foods fortified with B$_{12}$ or take a daily or weekly B$_{12}$ supplement. Fortified breakfast cereals are a particularly valuable source of vitamin B$_{12}$ for vegetarians and vegans. In addition, adults age 51 and older are recommended to consume B$_{12}$ fortified food or supplements to meet the RDA, because they are a population at an increased risk of deficiency.

Allergies

Vitamin B_{12} supplements in theory should be avoided in people sensitive or allergic to cobalamin, cobalt, or any other product ingredients. However, direct allergy to a vitamin or nutrient is extremely rare, and if reported, other causes should be sought.

Side effects, contraindications, and warnings

- Vitamin B_{12} has extremely low toxicity and even taking it in enormous doses appears not to be harmful to healthy individuals.
- Hematologic: Peripheral vascular thrombosis has been reported. Treatment of vitamin B_{12} deficiency can unmask polycythemia vera, which is characterized by an increase in blood volume and the number of red blood cells. The correction of megaloblastic anemia with vitamin B_{12} can result in fatal hypokalemia and gout in susceptible individuals, and it can obscure folate deficiency in megaloblastic anemia. Caution is warranted.
- Leber's disease: Vitamin B_{12} in the form of cyanocobalamin is contraindicated in early Leber's disease, which is hereditary optic nerve atrophy. Cyanocobalamin can cause severe and swift optic atrophy, but other forms of vitamin B_{12} are available.[citation needed] However, the sources of this statement are not clear, while an opposing view concludes: "The clinical picture of optic neuropathy associated with vitamin B_{12} deficiency shows similarity to that of Leber's disease optic neuropathy. Both involve the nerve fibres of the papillomacular bundle. The present case reports suggest that optic neuropathy in patients carrying a primary LHON mtDNA mutation may be precipitated by vitamin B_{12} deficiency. Therefore, known carriers should take care to have an adequate dietary intake of vitamin B_{12} and malabsorption syndromes like those occurring in familial pernicious anaemia or after gastric surgery should be excluded."

Other medical uses

Hydroxycobalamin, or hydoxocobalamin, also known as vitamin $B_{12}a$, is used in Europe both for vitamin B_{12} deficiency and as a treatment for cyanide poisoning, sometimes with a large amount (5–10 g) given intravenously, and sometimes in combination with sodium thiosulfate. The mechanism of action is straightforward: the hydroxycobalamin hydroxide ligand is displaced by the toxic cyanide ion, and the resulting harmless B_{12} complex is excreted in urine. In the United States, the Food and Drug Administration approved (in 2006) the use of hydroxocobalamin for acute treatment of cyanide poisoning.

High vitamin B_{12} level in elderly individuals may protect against brain atrophy or shrinkage, associated with Alzheimer's disease and impaired cognitive function.

Vitamin B_{12} enhances the phase-response of circadian melatonin rhythm to a single bright light exposure in humans. Sleep disturbances may occur because B_{12} may be involved in the regulation of the sleep wake cycle by the pineal gland (through melatonin).

Topical application of vitamin B_{12} has been shown to be an effective treatment for psoriasis.

Interactions

Interactions with drugs

- Alcohol (ethanol): Excessive alcohol intake lasting longer than two weeks can decrease vitamin B_{12} absorption from the gastrointestinal tract.[citation needed]

- Aminosalicylic acid (para-aminosalicylic acid, PAS, Paser): Aminosalicylic acid can reduce oral vitamin B_{12} absorption, possibly by as much as 55%, as part of a general malabsorption syndrome. Megaloblastic changes, and occasional cases of symptomatic anemia have occurred, usually after doses of 8 to 12 g/day for several months. Vitamin B_{12} levels should be monitored in people taking aminosalicylic acid for more than one month.

- Antibiotics: An increased bacterial load can bind significant amounts of vitamin B_{12} in the gut, preventing its absorption. In people with bacterial overgrowth of the small bowel, antibiotics such as metronidazole (Flagyl) can actually improve vitamin B_{12} status. The effects of most antibiotics on gastrointestinal bacteria are unlikely to have clinically significant effects on vitamin B_{12} levels.

- Hormonal contraception: The data regarding the effects of oral contraceptives on vitamin B_{12} serum levels are conflicting. Some studies have found reduced serum levels in oral contraceptive users, but others have found no effect despite use of oral contraceptives for up to 6 months. When oral contraceptive use is stopped, normalization of vitamin B_{12} levels usually occurs. Lower vitamin B_{12} serum levels seen with oral contraceptives probably are not clinically significant.

- Chloramphenicol (Chloromycetin): Limited case reports suggest that chloramphenicol can delay or interrupt the reticulocyte response to supplemental vitamin B_{12} in some patients. Blood counts should be monitored closely if this combination cannot be avoided.

- Cobalt irradiation: Cobalt irradiation of the small bowel can decrease gastrointestinal (GI) absorption of vitamin B_{12}.

- Colchicine: Colchicine in doses of 1.9 to 3.9 mg/day can disrupt normal intestinal mucosal function, leading to malabsorption of several nutrients, including vitamin B_{12}. Lower doses do not seem to have a significant effect on vitamin B_{12} absorption after 3 years of colchicine therapy. The significance of this interaction is unclear. Vitamin B_{12} levels should be monitored in people taking large doses of colchicine for prolonged periods.

- Colestipol (Colestid), cholestyramine (Questran): These resins used for sequestering bile acids to decrease cholesterol, can decrease gastrointestinal (GI) absorption of vitamin B_{12}. It is unlikely this interaction will deplete body stores of vitamin B_{12} unless there are other factors contributing to deficiency. In a group of children treated with cholestyramine for up to 2.5 years, there was not any change in serum vitamin B_{12} levels. Routine supplements are not necessary.

- H$_2$-receptor antagonists: include cimetidine (Tagamet), famotidine (Pepcid), nizatidine (Axid), and ranitidine (Zantac). Reduced secretion of gastric acid and pepsin produced by H$_2$ blockers can reduce absorption of protein-bound (dietary) vitamin B$_{12}$, but not of supplemental vitamin B$_{12}$. Gastric acid is needed to release vitamin B$_{12}$ from protein for absorption. Clinically significant vitamin B$_{12}$ deficiency and megaloblastic anemia are unlikely, unless H$_2$ blocker therapy is prolonged (2 years or more), or the person's diet is poor. It is also more likely if the person is rendered achlorhydric (with complete absence of gastric acid secretion), which occurs more frequently with proton pump inhibitors than H$_2$ blockers. Vitamin B$_{12}$ levels should be monitored in people taking high doses of H$_2$ blockers for prolonged periods.

- Metformin (Glucophage): Metformin may reduce serum folic acid and vitamin B$_{12}$ levels. These changes can lead to hyperhomocysteinemia, adding to the risk of cardiovascular disease in people with diabetes.[citation needed] There are also rare reports of megaloblastic anemia in people who have taken metformin for five years or more. Reduced serum levels of vitamin B$_{12}$ occur in up to 30% of people taking metformin chronically. However, clinically significant deficiency is not likely to develop if dietary intake of vitamin B$_{12}$ is adequate. Deficiency can be corrected with vitamin B$_{12}$ supplements even if metformin is continued. The metformin-induced malabsorption of vitamin B$_{12}$ is reversible by oral calcium supplementation. The general clinical significance of metformin upon B$_{12}$ levels is as yet unknown.

- Neomycin: Absorption of vitamin B$_{12}$ can be reduced by neomycin, but prolonged use of large doses is needed to induce pernicious anemia. Supplements are not usually needed with normal doses.

- Nicotine: Nicotine can reduce serum vitamin B$_{12}$ levels. The need for vitamin B$_{12}$ supplementation in smokers has not been adequately studied.

- Nitrous oxide: Nitrous oxide inactivates the cobalamin form of vitamin B$_{12}$ by oxidation. Symptoms of vitamin B$_{12}$ deficiency, including sensory neuropathy, myelopathy, and encephalopathy, can occur within days or weeks of exposure to nitrous oxide anesthesia in people with subclinical vitamin B$_{12}$ deficiency. Symptoms are treated with high doses of vitamin B$_{12}$, but recovery can be slow and incomplete. People with normal vitamin B$_{12}$ levels have sufficient vitamin B$_{12}$ stores to make the effects of nitrous oxide insignificant, unless exposure is repeated and prolonged (such as recreational use). Vitamin B$_{12}$ levels should be checked in people with risk factors for vitamin B$_{12}$ deficiency prior to using nitrous oxide anesthesia. Chronic nitrous oxide B$_{12}$ poisoning (usually from use of nitrous oxide as a recreational drug), however, may result in B$_{12}$ functional deficiency even with normal measured blood levels of B$_{12}$.

- Phenytoin (Dilantin), phenobarbital, primidone (Mysoline): These anticonvulsants have been associated with reduced vitamin B$_{12}$ absorption, and reduced serum and cerebrospinal fluid levels in some patients. This may contribute to the megaloblastic anemia, primarily caused by folate deficiency, associated with these drugs. It is also suggested that reduced vitamin B$_{12}$ levels may contribute to the neuropsychiatric side effects of these drugs. Patients should be encouraged to maintain adequate dietary vitamin B_{12} intake. Folate and vitamin B_{12} status should be checked if symptoms of anemia develop.

- Proton pump inhibitors (PPIs): The PPIs include omeprazole (Prilosec, Losec), lansoprazole (Prevacid), rabeprazole (Aciphex), pantoprazole (Protonix, Pantoloc), and esomeprazole (Nexium). The reduced secretion of gastric acid and pepsin produced by PPIs can reduce absorption of protein-bound (dietary) vitamin B_{12}, but not supplemental vitamin B_{12}. Gastric acid is needed to release vitamin B_{12} from protein for absorption. Reduced vitamin B_{12} levels may be more common with PPIs than with H2-blockers, because they are more likely to produce achlorhydria (complete absence of gastric acid secretion). However, clinically significant vitamin B_{12} deficiency is unlikely, unless PPI therapy is prolonged (2 years or more) or dietary vitamin intake is low. Vitamin B_{12} levels should be monitored in people taking high doses of PPIs for prolonged periods.
- Zidovudine (AZT, Combivir, Retrovir): Reduced serum vitamin B_{12} levels may occur when zidovudine therapy is started. This adds to other factors that cause low vitamin B_{12} levels in people with HIV, and might contribute to the hematological toxicity associated with zidovudine. However, the data suggest vitamin B_{12} supplements are not helpful for people taking zidovudine.

Interactions with herbs and dietary supplements

- Folic acid: Folic acid, particularly in large doses, can mask vitamin B_{12} deficiency by completely correcting hematological abnormalities. In vitamin B_{12} deficiency, folic acid can produce complete resolution of the characteristic megaloblastic anemia, while allowing potentially irreversible neurological damage (from continued inactivity of methylmalonyl mutase) to progress. Thus, vitamin B_{12} status should be determined before folic acid is given as monotherapy.
- Potassium: Potassium supplements can reduce absorption of vitamin B_{12} in some people. This effect has been reported with potassium chloride and, to a lesser extent, with potassium citrate. Potassium might contribute to vitamin B_{12} deficiency in some people with other risk factors, but routine supplements are not necessary.

See also

- Brachionus plicatilis
- Cobalamin
- Edible seaweed
- Pleurochrysis carterae

External links

- Vitamin B12 Fact Sheet [6] from the U.S. National Institutes of Health
- Jane Higdon, "Vitamin B12 [7]", Micronutrient Information Center, *Linus Pauling Institute*
- Vitamin B12 [8]. Medline Plus (National Library of Medicine). Part of it was used for this article (US Government public domain), specially for drug and other interactions.
- Vitamin B12 deficiency [9] article in *American Family Physician* journal
- MeSH *Cyanocobalamin* [10]
- Calculator for estimating the average daily Vitamin B12 intake [11]

Hydroxocobalamin

Hydroxocobalamin

Systematic (IUPAC) name	
Coα-[α-(5,6-dimethylbenzimidazolyl)]- Coβ-hydroxocobamide	
Identifiers	
CAS number	13422-51-0 [1]
ATC code	B03 BA03 [2] V03 AB33 [3]
PubChem	CID 6433575 [4]
DrugBank	APRD01022 [5]
ChemSpider	21160115 [6]
UNII	Q40X8H422O [7]
Chemical data	
Formula	$C_{64}H_{93}CoN_{13}O_{17}P$
Mol. mass	1406.46 g/mol
SMILES	eMolecules [8] & PubChem [9]
Pharmacokinetic data	
Protein binding	Very high (90%)
Metabolism	Primarily hepatic. Cobalamins are absorbed in the ileum and stored in the liver.
Half-life	~6 days
Therapeutic considerations	
Pregnancy cat.	?

Legal status	
Routes	Injectable (IM)

(what is this?) (verify) [10]

Hydroxocobalamin (OHCbl, or B_{12a}) is a natural form or vitamer of vitamin B_{12}, a basic member of the cobalamin family of compounds. Hydroxocobalamin is the form of vitamin B_{12} produced by many bacteria which are used to produce the vitamin commercially. Like other forms of vitamin B_{12}, hydroxocobalamin has an intense red color. It is not a form normally found in the human body, but is easily converted in the body to usable coenzyme forms of vitamin B_{12}. Pharmaceutically, hydroxycobalamin is usually produced as a sterile injectable solution, and is used for treatment of the vitamin deficiency, and also (because of its afinity for cyanide ion) as a treatment for cyanide poisoning.

Vitamin B_{12} is a term that refers to a group of compounds called cobalamins that are available in the human body in a variety of mostly interconvertible forms. Together with folic acid, cobalamins are essential cofactors required for DNA synthesis in cells where chromosomal replication and division are occurring—most notably the bone marrow and myeloid cells. As a cofactor, cobalamins are essential for two cellular reactions: (1) the mitochondrial methylmalonylcoenzyme A mutase conversion of methylmalonic acid (MMA) to succinate, which links lipid and carbohydrate metabolism, and (2) activation of methionine synthase, which is the rate limiting step in the synthesis of methionine from homocysteine and 5-methyltetrahydrofolate (Katzung, 1989).

Chemical characteristics

Description: OHCbl acetate occurs as an odorless, dark-red orthorhombic needles. The injection formulations appear as a clear, dark-red solution. Distribution Coefficient: 1.133×10-5 (octanol:acetate buffer pH 7.4) pKa: 7.65 Systematic Name: Cobinamide, Co-hydroxy-, dihydrogen phosphate (ester), inner salt, 3'- ester with (5,6-dimethyl-1-alpha-D-ribofuranosyl-1H-benzimidazole-kappaN3)

Causes of deficiency

Hydroxocobalamin Injection USP, are used to rectify the following causes of vitamin B_{12} deficiency (list taken from the drug prescription label published by the U.S. Food and Drug Administration (FDA):

- Pernicious anemia, whether uncomplicated or accompanied by nervous system involvement
- Dietary deficiency of vitamin B_{12} occurring in strict vegetarians and in their breastfed infants. (Isolated vitamin B_{12} deficiency is very rare.)
- Malabsorption of vitamin B_{12} resulting from structural or functional damage to the stomach where intrinsic factor is secreted or to the ileum where intrinsic factor facilitates vitamin B_{12} absorption (These conditions include tropical sprue and nontropical sprue [idiopathic steatorrhea, gluten-induced enteropathy]. Folate deficiency in these patients is usually more severe than vitamin B_{12} deficiency.)
- Inadequate secretion of intrinsic factor, resulting from lesions that destroy the gastric mucosa (ingestion of corrosives, extensive neoplasia, and a number of conditions associated with a variable degree of gastric atrophy, such as multiple sclerosis, certain endocrine disorders, iron deficiency, and subtotal gastrectomy). (Total gastrectomy always produces vitamin B_{12} deficiency.)
- Structural lesions leading to vitamin B_{12} deficiency include regional ileitis, ileal reactions, malignancies, etc.
- Competition for vitamin B_{12} by intestinal parasites or bacteria
- The fish tapeworm (*Diphyllobothrium latum*) absorbs huge quantities of vitamin B_{12} and infested patients often have associated gastric atrophy. The blind loop syndrome may produce deficiency of vitamin B_{12} or folate.
- Inadequate utilization of vitamin B_{12} (This may occur if antimetabolites for the vitamin are employed in the treatment of neoplasia.)

Indications

Vitamin B_{12} deficiency

Vitamin B_{12} compounds are used as prescription medicine (injection) for vitamin B_{12} replacement therapy, usually at 100 mcg/dose. In the UK 1,000mcg (1 mg) per dose is generally used. Damage that results from vitamin B_{12} deficiency can be prevented with early diagnosis and adequate treatment.

For most, the standard therapy for treatment of vitamin B_{12} deficiency has been intramuscular (IM) injections of vitamin B_{12} in the form of cyanocobalamin (CNCbl) or hydroxocobalamin (OHCbl). CNCbl is traditionally prescribed in the United States. Outside of the United States, OHCbl is most generally used for vitamin B_{12} replacement therapy and is considered the "drug of choice" for vitamin B_{12} deficiency by the Martindale Extra Pharmacopoeia (Sweetman, 2002) and the World Health Organization (WHO) Model List of Essential Drugs. This preference for OHCbl in many countries is due to its long retention in the body and the need for less frequent IM injections in restoring vitamin B_{12} (cobalamin) serum levels. Furthermore, IM administration of OHCbl is also the preferred treatment for pediatric patients with intrinsic cobalamin metabolic diseases; vitamin B_{12} deficient patients with tobacco amblyopia due to cyanide poisoning; and patients with pernicious anemia who have optic neuropathy (Carethers, 1988; Chisholm et al., 1967; Freeman, 1992; Markle, 1996).

In a newly-diagnosed vitamin B_{12}-deficient patient, normally defined as when serum cobalamin (vitamin B_{12}) levels are less than 200 pg/mL, daily IM injections of OHCbl up to 1,000 µg (1 mg) per day are given to replenish the body's depleted cobalamin stores. In the presence of neurological symptoms, following daily treatment, injections up to weekly or biweekly are indicated for 6 months before initiating monthly IM injections. Once clinical improvement is confirmed, maintenance supplementation of B_{12} will generally be needed for life.

Cyanide poisoning

Hydroxocobalamin has also been used in the treatment of cyanide poisoning.

Hydoxyocobalamin is marketed under the trade name Cyanokit for cyanide toxicity. The standard dose is 5g IV infused over 15 minutes. A second 5mg dose can be given in patients with severe toxicity. Hydroxocobalamin will bind circulating and cellular cyanide molecules to form cyanocobalamin which is excreted in the urine.

Toxicity

The literature data on the acute toxicity profile of OHCbl show that it is generally regarded as safe with local and systemic exposure. The ability of OHCbl to rapidly scavenge and detoxify cyanide by chelation has resulted in several acute animal and human studies using systemic OHCbl doses at suprapharmacological doses as high as 140 mg/kg to support its use as an intravenous (IV) treatment for cyanide exposure (Forsyth et al., 1993; Riou et al., 1993). The US FDA at the end of 2006 approved the use OHCbl as an injection for the treatment of cyanide poisoning.

Vitamin B_{12} group

Vitamin B_{12} is a term that refers to a group of compounds called cobalamins that are available in the human body in a variety of mostly interconvertible forms. Together with folic acid, cobalamins are essential cofactors required for DNA synthesis in cells where chromosomal replication and division are occurring—most notably the bone marrow and myeloid cells. As a cofactor, cobalamins are essential for two cellular reactions: (1) the mitochondrial methylmalonyl coenzyme A mutase conversion of methylmalonic acid (MMA) to succinate, which links lipid and carbohydrate metabolism, and (2) activation of methionine synthase, which is the rate limiting step in the synthesis of methionine from homocysteine and tetrahydrofolate (Katzung, 1989). Cobalamins are characterized by a porphyrin-like corrin nucleus that contains a single cobalt atom bound to a benzimidazolyl nucleotide and a variable residue (R) group. The variable R group gives rise to the four most commonly known cobalamins: CNCbl, methylcobalamin, 5-deoxyadenosylcobalamin, and OHCbl. In the serum, OHCbl and CNCbl are believed to function as storage or transport forms of the molecule; whereas, methylcobalamin and 5 deoxyadenosylcobalamin are the active forms of the coenzyme required for cell growth and replication (Katzung, 1989). CNCbl is usually converted to OHCbl in the serum, whereas OHCbl is converted to either methylcobalamin or 5 deoxyadenosyl cobalamin. Cobalamins circulate bound to serum proteins called transcobalamins (TC) and haptocorrins. OHCbl has a higher affinity to the TC II transport protein than CNCbl, or 5- deoxyadenosylcobalamin. From a biochemical point of view, two essential enzymatic reactions require vitamin B_{12} (cobalamin) (Katzung, 1989, Hardman, 2001). Intracellular vitamin B_{12} is maintained in two active coenzymes, methylcobalamin and 5 deoxyadenosylcobalamin, which are both involved in specific enzymatic reactions. In the face of vitamin B_{12} deficiency, conversion of methylmalonyl-CoA to succinyl-CoA cannot take place, which results in accumulation of methylmalonyl CoA and aberrant fatty acid synthesis. In the other enzymatic reaction, methylcobalamin supports the methionine synthase reaction, which is essential for normal metabolism of folate. The folate-cobalamin interaction is pivotal for normal synthesis of purines and pyrimidines and the transfer of the methyl group to cobalamin is essential for the adequate supply of tetrahydrofolate, the substrate for metabolic steps that require folate. In a state of vitamin B_{12} deficiency, the cell responds by redirecting folate metabolic pathways to supply increasing amounts of methyltetrahydrofolate. The resulting elevated concentrations of homocysteine and MMA are often found in patients with low serum vitamin B_{12} and can usually be lowered with successful vitamin B_{12} replacement therapy. However, elevated MMA and homocysteine concentrations may persist in patients with cobalamin concentrations between 200 to 350 pg/mL (Lindenbaum et al. 1994). Supplementation with vitamin B_{12} during conditions of deficiency restores the intracellular level of cobalamin and maintains a sufficient level of the two active coenzymes: methylcobalamin and deoxyadenosylcobalamin.

External links

- Hydroxocobalamin [11] in the ChEBI database

Cyanocobalamin

Cyanocobalamin	
Identifiers	
CAS number	68-19-9 [1]
PubChem	16212801 [2]
EC number	200-680-0 [3]
Properties	
Molecular formula	$C_{63}H_{88}CoN_{14}O_{14}P$
Molar mass	1355.38 g/mol
Appearance	Dark red solid
Melting point	> 300 °C
Boiling point	> 300 °C
Solubility in water	Soluble
Hazards	
MSDS	External MSDS from Fisher Scientific [4]
EU classification	Not available
S-phrases	S24/25
NFPA 704	
Flash point	N/A
Except where noted otherwise, data are given for materials in their standard state (at 25 °C, 100 kPa)	
Infobox references	

Cyanocobalamin is an especially common vitamer of the vitamin B_{12} family. It is the most famous vitamer of the family, because it is, in chemical terms, the most air-stable. It is the easiest to crystallize and, therefore, easiest to purify after it is produced by bacterial fermentation. A form of vitamin B_{12} called hydroxocobalamin is produced by bacteria, and then changed to cyanocobalamin in the process of being purified in activated charcoal columns after being separated from the bacterial cultures. Cyanide is naturally present in activated charcoal, and hydroxocobalamin, which has great affinity for cyanide, picks it up, and is changed to cyanocobalamin. Thus, the cyanocobalamin form of B_{12} is the most widespread in the food industry.

This fact has caused some people (usually from reading labels on packages and vitamin supplements, in which vitamin B_{12} is almost always listed last, since ingredients by law are listed in order of weight percentage), to infer that the correct chemical name of vitamin B_{12} actually *is* cyanocobalamin. In fact, vitamin B_{12} is the name for a whole class of chemicals with vitamin B_{12} activity, and cyanocobalamin is only one of these. Cyanocobalamin usually does not even occur in nature, and is not one of the forms of the vitamin that are directly used in the human body (or that of any other animal). However, animals and humans can convert cyanocobalamin to active (cofactor) forms of the vitamin, such as methylcobalamin. This process happens by equilibration, as cyanocobalamin slowly loses its cyanide in surroundings that contain no cyanide.[citation needed]

Cyanide is present in almost every type of smoke produced by burning organic materials, including tobacco and cannabis; therefore, there is some concernWikipedia:Avoid weasel words that vitamin B_{12}-deficient smokers should not be given cyanocobalamin, as it will have more difficulty being broken down.[citation needed] In such cases, other forms of vitamin B_{12} for injection (such as hydroxocobalamin itself) are commonly available as pharmaceuticals, and are actually the most commonly used injectable forms of vitamin B_{12} in many countries. Injectable cyanocobalamin remains the most commonly injectable vitamin B_{12} in the United States.

Chemical properties

Dark red crystals or an amorphous or crystalline red powder. Cyanocobalamin is very hygroscopic in the anhydrous form, and sparingly soluble in water (1:80). It is stable to autoclaving for short periods at 121 °C. The vitamin B_{12} coenzymes are very unstable in light.

The chemical name is 5,6-dimethyl-benzimidazolyl cyanocobamide.

Pharmaceutical use

Cyanocobalamin is usually prescribed for the following reasons: after surgical removal of part or all of the stomach or intestine to ensure there are adequate levels of vitamin B_{12} in the bloodstream; to treat pernicious anemia; vitamin B_{12} deficiency due to low intake from food; thyrotoxicosis; hemorrhage; malignancy; liver or kidney disease. Cyanocobalamin injections are often prescribed to gastric bypass patients having had part of their small intestine bypassed, making it difficult for B_{12} to be absorbed via food or vitamins. Cyanocobamide is also used to perform the Schilling test to check a person's ability to absorb vitamin B_{12}.

Possible side effects

The oral use of cyanocobalamin may lead to several allergic reactions such as hives; difficult breathing; swelling of the face, lips, tongue, or throat. Less-serious side effects may include headache, nausea, stomach upset, diarrhea, joint pain, itching, or rash.

In the treatment of some forms of anemia (e.g., megaloblastic anemia), the use of cyanocobalamin can lead to severe hypokalemia, sometimes fatal, due to intracellular potassium shift upon anemia resolution. When treated with vitamin B_{12}, patients with Leber's disease may suffer rapid optic atrophy.[citation needed]

Article Sources and Contributors

Pernicious anemia *Source*: http://en.wikipedia.org/?oldid=387799592 *Contributors*:

Hypertension *Source*: http://en.wikipedia.org/?oldid=390483525 *Contributors*: MrOllie

Hypotension *Source*: http://en.wikipedia.org/?oldid=390483639 *Contributors*: MrOllie

Fatigue (medical) *Source*: http://en.wikipedia.org/?oldid=390156433 *Contributors*: Berean Hunter

Tachycardia *Source*: http://en.wikipedia.org/?oldid=390021779 *Contributors*: Jmh649

Pallor *Source*: http://en.wikipedia.org/?oldid=388558961 *Contributors*: 1 anonymous edits

Depression (mood) *Source*: http://en.wikipedia.org/?oldid=390500905 *Contributors*: MrOllie

Weakness *Source*: http://en.wikipedia.org/?oldid=390260950 *Contributors*:

Dyspnea *Source*: http://en.wikipedia.org/?oldid=390044893 *Contributors*: Jmh649

Neuropathic pain *Source*: http://en.wikipedia.org/?oldid=389461164 *Contributors*: Picardlm

Diarrhea *Source*: http://en.wikipedia.org/?oldid=387664528 *Contributors*: LordMaster96

Paresthesia *Source*: http://en.wikipedia.org/?oldid=390365230 *Contributors*: 1 anonymous edits

Jaundice *Source*: http://en.wikipedia.org/?oldid=390236197 *Contributors*:

Glossitis *Source*: http://en.wikipedia.org/?oldid=362421337 *Contributors*: Gobonobo

Atrophic gastritis *Source*: http://en.wikipedia.org/?oldid=377910391 *Contributors*: 1 anonymous edits

Helicobacter pylori *Source*: http://en.wikipedia.org/?oldid=389263888 *Contributors*: 1 anonymous edits

Complete blood count *Source*: http://en.wikipedia.org/?oldid=390619759 *Contributors*: 1 anonymous edits

Schilling test *Source*: http://en.wikipedia.org/?oldid=362437615 *Contributors*: Gobonobo

Diphyllobothrium *Source*: http://en.wikipedia.org/?oldid=390161785 *Contributors*:

Vitamin B *Source*: http://en.wikipedia.org/?oldid=390380752 *Contributors*: Ahoerstemeier

Hydroxocobalamin *Source*: http://en.wikipedia.org/?oldid=390495858 *Contributors*:

Cyanocobalamin *Source*: http://en.wikipedia.org/?oldid=386955872 *Contributors*: Edgar181

Image Sources, Licenses and Contributors

CPSIA information can be obtained at www.ICGtesting.com
Printed in the USA
LVOW112307280213

322207LV00003B/71/P